HANDBOOK *of*
GLOBAL MENTAL HEALTH

FIRST EDITION

I0106240

SARA ANNE SPOWART, PhD, LMFT

Copyright ©2024 by Sara Anne Spowart, PhD, LMFT.

ISBN 978-1-964097-56-5 (softcover)
ISBN 978-1-964097-57-2 (ebook)

All rights reserved. No part of this book may be reproduced or transmitted in any form or by any means, electronic or mechanical, including photocopying, recording, or by any information storage and retrieval system without express written permission from the author, except in the case of brief quotations embodied in critical reviews and certain other non-commercial uses permitted by copyright law.

Printed in the United States of America.

HANDBOOK *of* GLOBAL MENTAL HEALTH

—— FIRST EDITION ——

SARA ANNE SPOWART, PhD, LMFT

TABLE OF CONTENTS

CHAPTER 1. **OVERVIEW AND BACKGROUND ON THE SIGNIFICANCE OF GLOBAL MENTAL HEALTH**   **1**

Introduction...1

Key Terms and Definitions 1

  Happiness *1*

  Depression *2*

  Purpose *2*

  Mindfulness *2*

  Connection *2*

  Mental Health *2*

Overview of Mental Health and Well-Being..3

Inadequacy of Mental Health Treatment...3

  Significance of Mental Health Facts *3*

Significance of Mental Health Worldwide: Depression 4

Significance of Mental Health Worldwide: Population..4

Significance of Mental Health Worldwide: Anxiety..4

Significance of Mental Health Worldwide: Population Impact...5

Significance of Mental Health Worldwide: Holistic Approach 6

  Mental Health Is Important *6*

The Rising Importance of Mental Health Treatment Worldwide......................................7

The Mental Health Treatment Gap 8

Evolution of Mental Health Treatment 8

Child Mental Health, Prevention, and Treatment 9

List of Key Takeaways..10

Review Questions...11

References 12

CHAPTER 2. **OVERVIEW AND BACKGROUND ON TREATMENT OF MENTAL HEALTH**   **13**

Introduction..13

Key Terms and Definitions 13

  Mental Health Stigma *13*

  Mental Health Literacy *13*

  Evidence-Based Therapy *14*

  Mental Health First Aid *14*

  Overview of Treatment of Mental Health *14*

Mental Health Stigma 15

Mental Health Literacy..16

Mental Health First Aid...17

Solution-Focused Therapy 17

Cognitive Behavior Therapy 18

Rational Emotive Behavior Therapy 19

Group Support and Group Therapy 20

Yoga 20

Family Therapy..21

List of Key Takeaways..21

Review Questions...21

References 22

CHAPTER 3. **MENTAL HEALTH, TREATMENT, AND HAPPINESS IN LATIN AMERICA**   **23**
   Introduction 23
   Key Terms and Definitions 23
        Latin America 23
        The Caracas Declaration 24
        Crime Victimization 24
        Underrepresented Groups in Latin America 24
        The Latin American Paradox 24
        Overview and Background of Mental Health in Latin America 25

   History of Latin American Region and Well-Being 25
   Latin America and Happiness 26
   The Anomaly of Latin American Well-Being 27
   Latin America and Mental Illness 27
   Mental Health Investment in Latin America 28
   The Caracas Declaration and Latin American Mental Health 28
   Crime Victimization in Latin America 29
        Growth of Crime in Latin America 29
        Paradox of Crime, Victimization, and Well-Being 30

   Barriers to Mental Health Care and Well-Being in Latin America 30
   Innovative Approaches for Mental Health Treatment in Latin America 30
   Mental Health of Underrepresented Groups in Latin America 32
        LGBTQ Groups and Mental Health in Latin America 32
        Criminal Offenders and Mental Health in Latin America 32

   Rural Low-Income Groups and Mental Health in Latin America 33
   Indigenous Groups and Mental Health in Latin America 33
   Summary 34
   List of Key Takeaways 34
   Review Questions 34
   References 35

CHAPTER 4. **OVERVIEW OF VARIATION IN MENTAL ILLNESS AND TREATMENT IN EUROPE**   **36**
   Introduction 36
   Key Terms and Definitions 36
        "Nordic Exceptionalism" 36
        European Mental Health Action Plan 37
        Late Life Depression 37
        Overview and Background on Mental Illness, Happiness, and Treatment in Europe 37

   European Mental Health and Treatment 38
   World Health Organization and the Significance of Mental Health in Europe 39
   The Prevalence of Late-Life Depression in Europe 40
   The Treatment Gap in Europe 41
   COVID, Mental Health, and Happiness in Europe 42
   Case Study of Italy with COVID 42
        Solutions Resulting from the Italy Case Study 43

   Tele-Psychotherapy 43
   Improved Healthcare and Social Support for the Mentally Ill 44
   Mental Health Progress in Europe 44
   Child Mental Illness 45
   Prevention 45
   List of Key Takeaways 46
   Review Questions 46
   References 47

CHAPTER 5. **MENTAL HEALTH IN SUB-SAHARAN AFRICA** **48**
Introduction...48
Key Terms and Definitions...48
    Sub-Saharan African Optimism.. 48
    Happiness Deficit 49
    Resilience 49
    Overview 49

Mental Health and Treatment in Sub-Saharan Africa...50
    Research Challenges.. 50
    The Gallup World Poll and Hadley Cantril.................................. 51
    Lived Poverty and Happiness... 51
    The Case of South Africa... 52
    The Rise of Technology and Current Trends................................. 52
    Adolescent Mental Health and Happiness................................... 53

The Growth of Identified Mental Illness in Sub-Saharan Africa 54
    Access to Treatment... 54
    Resiliency and Protective Factors.. 55
    Recent Changes in Mental Health in Sub-Saharan Africa 56

List of Key Takeaways...58
Review Questions..58
References 59

CHAPTER 6. **MENTAL HEALTH AND HAPPINESS IN ASIA** **61**
Introduction...61
Key Terms and Definitions...61
    Microfinance... 61
    REACH 62
    Mobile Health... 62
    Gross National Happiness (GNH) 62
    Overview 63

The Importance of Mental Health 63
The Importance of Mental Health in South Asia...63
Mental Health and Youth in Asia..64
Positive Strengths of Mental Health in Asia: Family, Love, and Mental Health 65
Positive Strengths of Mental Health in Asia: The Importance of Ritual..................................65
Challenges of Mental Health in Asia: Natural Disasters..66
Challenges of Mental Health in Asia: Mental Health Stigma 66
Case Study: Mental Health and Treatment in China...67
Changes in Happiness Rankings in China...67
Case Study: Mental Health in Bhutan..69
Mental Health Innovations: Mobile Health..69
Mental Health Innovations: Microfinance in Asia...70
Conclusion..71
List of Key Takeaways...71
Review Questions..71
References 72

CHAPTER 7. **MENTAL HEALTH IN THE UNITED STATES**   **73**
Introduction...73
Key Terms and Definitions..73
    The United States Happiness Paradox 73
    DACA 73
    The Great Recession 74
    Happiness Inequality 74
    Overview 74

Mental Health in the United States and Treatment..74
    Overview on U.S. Mental Health. 74
    The United States Happiness Paradox 75
    United States and the Great Recession. 76
    Five Significant Factors in United States Happiness 76
    The United States and Social and Family Connections 77
    Happiness Inequality in the United States 77

Unique Aspects of Happiness and Well-Being in the United States..78
    Longevity and Happiness in the United States 78
    Volunteering and Happiness in the United States. 79
    Gun Ownership and Happiness in the United States 79

Mental Health and the University in the United States...79
COVID and Well-Being in the United States...80
Immigrant Inequality..80
Conclusion...81
List of Key Takeaways...81
Review Questions...81
References..82

CHAPTER 8. **THE IMPACT OF THE GLOBAL TREATMENT GAP**   **83**
Introduction...83
Key Terms and Definitions..83
    Mental Health Protective Factors 83
    Overdose Epidemic 83
    Unconditional Positive Regard 84
    Overview 84

The Impact of Mental Illness..84
    Inadequacy of Mental Health Treatment. 84

Overview of Previous Chapters..85
    Population Impact. 85

The Rising Importance of Mental Health Treatment Worldwide 86
The Impact of the European Treatment Gap...86
The Impact of the African Treatment Gap..87
The Impact of the United States Treatment Gap...87
Factors that Create, Maintain, or Grow the Mental Health Treatment Gap 88
    Mental Health Stigma. 88
    Mental Health Literacy 88
    Lack of Early Identification 89
    Lack of Political Will, Funding, and Focus 89

Pre-Existing Protective Factors for Mental Health...89
    The Case of Latin America. 89
    The Case of Asia 90
    Cultural Protective Factors 90
    Mobile Health. 91
    Family and Relational Support. 91
    The Use of Ritual. 92
    The Case of The United States. 92
    Volunteering 92

Conclusion...92
List of Key Takeaways...93
Review Questions...93
References..94

CHAPTER 9. **THE FUTURE OF MENTAL HEALTH TREATMENT** **96**

Introduction...96
Key Terms and Definitions..97
    Solution-Focused Therapy...................................... *97*
    E-health.. *97*
    Public Health Campaigns...................................... *97*
    Overview... *97*

Mental Health Progress...98
The Future and Child Mental Health..98
    Intervention Approach... *99*
    Overcoming Mental Health Stigma......................... *99*

Effective Interventions for the Future of Mental Health 99
    Mental Health First Aid....................................... *99*
    Solution-Focused Therapy...................................... *100*
    Cognitive Behavior Therapy.................................. *101*
    Rational Emotive Behavior Therapy........................ *101*
    Group Support and Group Therapy......................... *101*
    Yoga.. *102*
    Family Therapy.. *102*
    Latin America and E-Health.................................. *102*
    Prevention.. *102*

Conclusion...103
List of Key Takeaways..103
Review Questions..103
References...104

CHAPTER 1

OVERVIEW AND BACKGROUND ON THE SIGNIFICANCE OF GLOBAL MENTAL HEALTH

"Mental health can be just as important as physical health – and major depression is one of the most commonly diagnosed mental illnesses."
—Michael Greger

INTRODUCTION

This chapter provides an overview of the importance of global mental health as well as the evolution and rise of its importance worldwide. It also includes relevant World Health Organization information on predictions for depression, suicidal ideation, and mental illness as leading global illnesses. As a rising issue of concern, it is important to learn more about the basics of global mental health and some generally effective approaches to treatment. Working knowledge of global mental health is relevant and significant for numerous areas of comprehension.

KEY TERMS AND DEFINITIONS

Below are common definitions and key terms that will be addressed and used throughout this book.

Happiness

- Happiness is characterized as a state of contentment and overall satisfaction with one's current situation. It can be measured by subjective quantitative and qualitative interpretations.
- Happiness is a temporary state. However, the characteristics that comprise happiness such as a sense of purpose, connection, meaning, and working towards a higher purpose than oneself are more stable and long-lasting.
- Happiness may require ongoing improvements in the characteristics that comprise it to maintain a certain level of well-being (Baumeister et al., 2013; Kim-Prieto et al., 2005).

1

Depression

- Depression is a state characterized by feelings of sadness and/or loss of interest in activities one typically enjoys.
- Depression can lead to a mix of mental and physical health concerns and impair one's ability to function in everyday life at work, at home, and in relationships.
- In addition, it can be characterized by fatigue, agitation, feelings of worthlessness, thoughts of death or suicide, difficulty concentrating, and changes in appetite (Bernard, 2018).

Purpose

- Purpose is the ongoing intention to accomplish a long-term goal that is meaningful on a personal level as well as contributes something positive to the greater good.
- An individual's perspective on purpose can change over the life course and evolve as goals are achieved. Purpose is not an abiding state but everchanging and can be short lived. It is not a constant and is not necessarily a permanent experience (George & Park, 2013).

Mindfulness

- Mindfulness is the practice of intentionally bringing one's attention to the present moment without judgment.
- Mindfulness can be practiced through meditation and other trainings that help bring one's attention to the present moment.
- Increasing one's level of mindfulness may impact one's interpretation and understanding of their happiness levels (Anālayo, 2019).

Connection

- Connection is the relationship an individual or thing has with something else and the association between them. It is the linking of one thing with another.
- Connection can occur from a feeling of love and engagement with people, places, things, and ideas that are deemed important and of interest (Klussman et al., 2022).

Mental Health

- According to the World Health Organization, mental health relates to mental and psychological well-being. It refers to emotional, psychological, and social well-being.
- Mental health impacts our inner state of well-being and can negatively impact our physical health. It is significant for every stage of life, from childhood through adulthood into older age. Our state of mental health impacts how we have relationships, manage stress, and make decisions (World Health Organization, 2017).

OVERVIEW OF MENTAL HEALTH AND WELL-BEING

At present, 94 countries, or 48% of all WHO member states have worked on their policies for mental health in line with international and regional human rights standards. These countries have either newly created or updated laws to include mental health as a significant factor that should be considered by global health rights standards (World Health Organization, 2017).

INADEQUACY OF MENTAL HEALTH TREATMENT

At present and worldwide, the amount of public expenditure that goes to mental health is very small and inadequate in low- and middle-income countries. The number of mental health workers is largely inadequate across the world. There are an estimated 72 mental health workers per 100,000 population in high-income countries and 1 mental health worker per 100,000 population in low-income countries. The global median number of mental health workers per 100,000 is 9, but there is major variation between low- and high-income countries for access and type of treatment. But in both high-income and low-income countries, mental health treatment is inadequately provided. Furthermore, more than 80% of this public expenditure is directed to funding mental health hospitals and not regular outpatient treatment. Mental health hospitals address the most acute, short-term mental health concerns and do not work in the community for prevention and treatment. This is a reactive, high-cost approach that increases the chance of disability due to mental illness. It is inadequate for reducing mental health issues on a wider scale for a greater range of mental health conditions in a country (Helliwell et al., 2018; WHO, 2021).

As of 2020, 72% of World Health Organization member states have an independent national mental health plan or policy, and 57% of member states have a stand-alone mental health law. Mental health is on the forefront of concerns being addressed by WHO member states. As of 2020, 62% of WHO member states have been modernizing their mental health policy and plan, and 40% have worked on revising their mental health law to better serve and address growing mental health concerns. Approximately 63% of WHO member states or 123 countries have a minimum of two functioning national, multisectoral mental health promotion and prevention programs. This is a great start but is still inadequate to address global health care needs (WHO, 2021).

Significance of Mental Health Facts

As you read the section below, please consider the implications and importance that mental health plays and how depression, anxiety, and suicide are not just mental health problems, but also general health concerns.

- Depression is the leading cause of disability worldwide.
- The number of individuals living with depression in 2017 was approximately 322 million people (4.4% of the world's population).
- The highest levels of depression occur on average worldwide from age 60–64 years.

- Over 800,000 people committed suicide in 2017, according to WHO.
- Anxiety is another significant mental health concern and often co-occurs with depression.
- Anxiety and depression rates are higher in low- and middle-income countries, although unusually high in the United States (a high-income country).
- Anxiety is the *6th* largest cause of disability in the world.
- Mental health concerns generally begin during adolescence.

SIGNIFICANCE OF MENTAL HEALTH WORLDWIDE: DEPRESSION

According to the American Medical Association, depression is the leading cause of disability in the world. Depression can express itself through a loss of interest in things that used to bring joy, low levels of motivation, changes in appetite and sleep, difficulty concentrating, low levels of energy and lethargy, anger or irritability, and suicidal ideation. Depression can be the result of a sense of hopelessness, of feeling stuck and not having power and control over one's life. It can also be the result of a combination of social, psychological, and biological factors. There are effective treatments for depression for individuals who are able to access assistance and are open to support. Some of these treatments include cognitive behavioral therapy, interpersonal mental health therapy, and medications such as antidepressants (Clark et al., 2017; Helliwell et al., 2017).

SIGNIFICANCE OF MENTAL HEALTH WORLDWIDE: POPULATION

In 2017, the number of individuals living with depression was estimated to be 322 million people or 4.4% of the world's population. It is more common with females (5.1%) than with males (3.6%). Depression levels are highest among women in the African region. Rates of depression are highest in older adulthood, specifically 55–74 years of age. Rates of depression are highest in the world among females in the African region and the Americas with the greatest prevalence of depression from age 60–64 years. The World Health Organization reported that the percentage of people living with depression increased by 18% from 2005–2015. The prevalence rates seem to peak in adults around 60 years of age, but this is also seen at heightened levels with teenagers. Without treatment, symptoms tend to worsen throughout the life span with each bout of depression. It can become a serious health condition and can lead to suicide. In 2017, WHO reported that over 800,000 people commit suicide every year. A large number of these are youth between the ages of 15–29 years (Clark et al., 2017; Helliwell et al., 2017; WHO, 2017).

SIGNIFICANCE OF MENTAL HEALTH WORLDWIDE: ANXIETY

Another prevalent and significant health concern is anxiety. Anxiety is the experience of apprehension, uneasiness, and nervousness over an anticipated or potential future event. It can be characterized by feelings of tension, worried thoughts, and physical sensations such as tense muscles, sweating, and increased blood pressure. It is a reaction to a perceived or real traumatic, stressful, or dangerous situation.

Anxiety often co-occurs with depression and significantly impacts levels of disability (WHO, 2017). The 2017 *World Happiness Report* stated that 260 million people or 3.6% of the global population suffer from anxiety (Helliwell et al., 2017). The prevalence of both anxiety and depression is actually higher in low- and middle-income countries than in high-income countries. However, there is variation in this with the United States being a high-income country with unusually high levels of mental illness. Here, anxiety includes conditions such as post-traumatic stress disorder, obsessive-compulsive disorders, panic disorder, and generalized anxiety disorder. These conditions increased by 14.9% globally from 2005 to 2015, and this was especially high in North America. In 2017, anxiety disorders were the 6th largest cause of disability in the world, and, like depression, more women are affected by anxiety disorders than men (Clark et al., 2017; Helliwell et al., 2017; WHO, 2017).

SIGNIFICANCE OF MENTAL HEALTH WORLDWIDE: POPULATION IMPACT

The majority of individuals suffering from depression and anxiety include women, young people, and the elderly. Anxiety disorders are more common in females (4.6%) than in males (2.6%) globally. In North America close to 8% of females are estimated to suffer from anxiety disorders. There was approximately a 15% increase in anxiety disorders from 2005 to 2015 worldwide due to aging and population growth. Many individuals experience anxiety and depression together as comorbidities. It is estimated that one-third of symptomatic cases follow a moderate-severe course (WHO, 2017). Depression is a major contributor to suicide. Depression is ranked as the single largest contributor to years of life disability or nonfatal health loss worldwide. In 2015, close to 800,000 people died due to suicide. However, an unknown and much greater number attempted but did not die by suicide. In 2015, suicide was in the top 20 causes of death, accounting for 1.5% of all deaths worldwide. It was the second leading cause of death among 15- to 29-year-old adolescents and adults. Females are more likely to suffer from suicidal ideation and suicide attempts but less likely to succeed in a suicide attempt. Males are more likely to succeed at a suicide attempt. Low- and middle-income countries experienced close to 80% of all suicides in 2015 (Clark et al., 2017; Helliwell et al., 2017; WHO, 2017).

These numbers and this report occurred before the COVID-19 pandemic when depression was already considered a leading cause of disability, and COVID greatly exasperated an already pre-existing issue and concern concerning mental illness. The issue of mental health is only of greater concern today with rates of mental illness significantly higher now than in 2015 and 2017. The real numbers for depression, and anxiety. and suicidal ideation are likely much higher than what is provided above. Our ability to account for the percentage of individuals living with mental illness worldwide is limited and also based on the willingness of individuals to report honestly and to understand what they are experiencing. Increased access to education and resources for depression, anxiety, and suicidal ideation, as well as more open conversations and reduced stigma, is important for increasing awareness and obtaining the most accurate data possible (Clark et al., 2017; Helliwell et al., 2017; WHO, 2017).

Mental disorders are a leading cause of disability worldwide. The onset of mental health disorders most often occurs during adolescence. A study conducted by Biswas and colleagues from the Global School-based Student

Health Survey (GSHS) on the prevalence of anxiety and suicidal ideation in a large worldwide population of adolescents in 82 countries reported that 14% suffered from suicidal ideation and 9% from anxiety (Biswas et al., 2020). These data demonstrate that mental health, specifically suicidal ideation, and anxiety, is a significant public health concern. The United Nations High Commissioner for Human Rights promotes and advocates for a rights-based approach to suicide prevention. Suicide is the second leading cause of death among adolescents, and numerous countries have reported increases in self-harm in recent years. However, in previous years, population-based studies have neglected to assess suicidal thoughts and behavior (Clark et al., 2017; Helliwell et al., 2017; WHO, 2017).

SIGNIFICANCE OF MENTAL HEALTH WORLDWIDE: HOLISTIC APPROACH

The United Nations High Commissioner is requesting a more holistic approach for individuals and populations as a whole that addresses the structural and psychosocial determinants of distress. The most recent research related to this has found that peer relationships, peer conflict, victimization, and isolation are all significant relational factors regarding adolescent anxiety and suicidal ideation. This supports research that shows associations among bullying, victimization, and suicidal thoughts and behaviors. Also, it was found that high levels of parental control were associated with poorer mental health and higher levels of parental understanding and monitoring were associated with better mental health in adolescents (Clark et al., 2017; Helliwell et al., 2017; WHO, 2017).

This data point to the importance of family-oriented interventions and practices for the treatment of youth mental health. Aside from family-oriented interventions, evidence indicates that school-based programs with universal mental health awareness are effective in addressing suicidal ideation and anxiety levels. However, implementing this on a large scale is challenging, and access is a notable barrier. However, the majority of evidence for these interventions is from high-income countries, although 75% of global suicides come from low- and middle-income countries, and youth are close to half the population in these countries. Therefore, research on young people in low- to middle-income countries is a significant research priority (Clark et al., 2017; Helliwell et al., 2017; WHO, 2017).

Mental Health Is Important

As you read the section below, please consider the importance of mental health on a larger scale and how population-wide interventions can potentially make a positive difference.

- At least 1 in 10 people suffer from mental illness at any time worldwide.
- More women than men suffer from both anxiety and depression worldwide. This may in part be due to gender inequality norms that lessen women's power and position in society.
- There is a significant treatment gap globally between mental health needs and actual services provided.

- Innovative, widespread programs such as Improving Access to Psychological Therapies (IAPT) in the United Kingdom have been significant for understanding the positive impact that easily accessible mental health programs can make on a population-wide basis.

THE RISING IMPORTANCE OF MENTAL HEALTH TREATMENT WORLDWIDE

Mental illness is a worldwide health phenomenon. Mental illness does not only occur in wealthy countries as has been stereotypically believed. The most recent data demonstrate that the vast majority of individuals with mental illness live in low- and middle-income regions of the world. The majority of these conditions relate to anxiety and depression disorders. In 2013, at least 1 in 10 people suffered globally from these conditions at any one time. These numbers are only higher today. Furthermore, the 2013 statistic is likely to be lower than the actual prevalence rates given the stigma and cultural considerations in reporting, understanding of mental illness, and availability of access to data (Helliwell & Wang, 2013; Layard et al., 2013).

Child and adolescent behavior and mental health issues further contribute to prevalence rates with an additional estimated 100 million cases worldwide. Prevalence rates are different among countries, but there is much less variation when groups of countries are clustered together by income level. In 2013, WHO estimated that 7.1% of adults in high-income countries suffered from depression, 7.6% in upper-middle income, 6.4% in lower-middle income, and 6% in low income. The data also reflect that among those with depression, there is a much higher number of women than men. Depression represents the greatest disability factor, according to WHO. The data have been further supportive in identifying a relationship between mental illness and national levels of happiness. In Western, Eastern, and Central Europe, those who suffer from anxiety and depression experience 12–14 years of lived disability due to their condition (Helliwell & Wang, 2013; Layard et al., 2013).

A major consideration in the incredible burden of mental illness is the lack of adequate mental health care and treatment for those who are suffering. There is a significant worldwide treatment gap between identified needs and actual service provision. In 2013, the treatment gap for schizophrenia, for example, was approximately 32%. However, even more telling, for all other conditions including more commonly identified issues such as anxiety, depression, and alcohol dependence, the treatment gap was greater than 50%. Worse than this, even when disability due to mental illness is severe, the treatment gap is still very significant. In 2013, only 10–30% of severe cases received services in low- and middle-income countries compared to 25–60% in high-income regions. The countries with the highest rates of treatment services included the United States, Spain, and Belgium for severe, moderate, and mild mental illness (Helliwell & Wang, 2013; Layard et al., 2013).

THE MENTAL HEALTH TREATMENT GAP

This treatment gap has severe consequences for society. Untreated mental illness creates major costs to society that come not only in monetary form but also through strained use of the healthcare system, lost productivity, educational underachievement, increased levels of violence, addiction, crime, less effective use of resources, breakdown of social and family relationships, worsening physical health and obesity, and lower overall development of human and societal potential. Treatment for mental illness has important implications for life expectancy, quality of life, and the burden of disability. For example, admittance to the hospital for mental health reasons improves life expectancy by an estimated 15–20 years (Helliwell & Wang, 2013; Layard et al., 2013).

Despite its demonstrated significance for health, economic, and societal outcomes, no country in the world spends more than 15% of its health budget on mental healthcare. The outliers that spend closest to 15% include England and Wales, and they have witnessed significant improvements in years and cost due to disability as a result of increased access and use of mental health services and government financing. There are low-cost and effective mental health treatments available that can be made much more widely available. It is harmful not to adequately incorporate mental health into a country's budget when there is so much evidence of harm for lack of treatment. Also, there are so many positive impacts on numerous quantifiers for development and wealth when mental health treatment is incorporated (Helliwell & Wang, 2013; Layard et al., 2013).

EVOLUTION OF MENTAL HEALTH TREATMENT

The field of mental healthcare has progressed significantly since the 1950s when the treatments available were extremely limited and torn between kind, compassionate care and more draconian residential psychiatric ward treatments. However, since the 1950s, significant breakthroughs have been made through new medications that help with depression, anxiety, bipolar, and psychotic disorders. In the 1970s, new evidenced-based therapy interventions were created including cognitive behavior therapy (CBT). It was discovered in the 1970s that up to 16 CBT sessions created similar recovery rates to medication, with lower relapse than medication (Helliwell & Wang, 2013 Layard et al., 2013).

With anxiety disorders, treatment with CBT and medication provides recovery rates of more than 50%. Therapy and drug interventions are inexpensive compared with treatment and intervention for a majority of individuals living with physical illness. When the larger cost of disability is considered, increasing wider access to psychological therapy reduces the gross cost for the public sector to zero. The research shows that there is no downside to increasing and expanding access to mental health treatment. If it reduces the level of disability, addiction, obesity, crime, relationship deterioration, unemployment, violence, and more, it will eventually add up to increased wealth and development for any country. This includes high-, middle-, and low-income regions (Helliwell & Wang, 2013; Layard et al., 2013).

This data and the understanding of the importance of mental health treatment and the overall positive impact it will have not only on society but on economics led the British government to conduct a novel program in 2008 until present to increase access to therapy. This program is called Improving Access to Psychological

Therapies (IAPT) and was an innovative and impressive initiative that the government took, based on sound data and evidence (Helliwell & Wang, 2013). As of 2013, the program served more than half a million people a year and continues to expand. The outcomes and rates of recovery are seen to be similar to that of clinical trials. These recovery rates are also reflected in these individuals being able to consistently maintain employment and not go on government disability (Helliwell & Wang, 2013; Layard et al., 2013).

The success of Britain's expanded government-backed therapy initiative IAPT helped Chile to consider implementing a similar program. In Chile, research on the cost and impact of depression treatment led to its incorporation and prioritization in the national health care program. Depression is now being considered a significant health problem when in the past it was not. Two separate studies that investigated the impacts of increased mental healthcare in India and the South-East Asia region found that depression treatment as defined by the two studies, created a minimum of 20 disability-free days in each region. Additional research also shows that providing a minimum of 10 sessions of CBT treatment also significantly increased the level of output per individual. Therefore, it was not only a consideration of less disability per day and lower costs to society, but also of higher and greater output levels (Helliwell & Wang, 2013; Layard et al., 2013).

CHILD MENTAL HEALTH, PREVENTION, AND TREATMENT

Aside from expanded access and lower cost of mental health services, another important consideration to reduce the burden of mental illness is addressing child mental illness. At least 50% of child mental illness is expressed by age 15. Child mental illness can be understood as the internalizing disorders that express themselves through anxiety and depression and externalizing disorders with behavior issues such as conduct disorder and attention-deficit hyperactivity disorder (ADHD). The evidence from clinical trials and larger government initiatives demonstrates that anxiety has 50–60% recovery rates with psychological therapy. Depression is effectively treated with CBT, interpersonal therapy, and medication with significant success rates. Conduct disorder when mild to moderate in severity and with parent training is treatable, and ADHD has a 70% recovery rate with the psychostimulant medication Methylphenidate. The data clearly demonstrate that early treatment with children is very effective as well as economically intelligent (Helliwell et al., 2015; Layard & Hagell, 2015).

Another component of this is not only early treatment but also prevention. By preventing the main risk factors that lead to mental illness, we can reduce the overall burden on society and the need to significantly expand treatment. The individual attributes that put one at risk for mental illness include low self-esteem, emotional immaturity, trouble with communication, medical illness, and substance abuse. Social circumstances that put one at risk for mental illness include loneliness, bereavement, neglect, family conflict, exposure to violence/abuse, low income and poverty, difficulties or failure at school, and work stress or unemployment.

Environmental factors that significantly impact mental health include poor access to basic services, injustice and discrimination, and exposure to war or disaster. Any or all combinations of these can lead to the development of mental illness in an individual. Early intervention programs and mental health initiatives serve as protective or preventive factors in developing mental illness (Helliwell et al., 2015; Layard & Hagell, 2015).

Some interventions can be conducted by community members through psychoeducational interventions for pregnant mothers and parents with young children. Interventions that are implemented in home, work, community, and school-based environments are effective for addressing needs. The stigma and misunderstanding about mental health may preclude individuals from accessing or trying to access mental health services aside from limitations in service provision and cost. This psychosocial support through education and public health measures may be an effective method to address multiple variables that put an individual at risk for developing a mental illness or learning how to manage early symptoms (Helliwell et al., 2015; Layard & Hagell, 2015).

At its core, the greatest issue with mental health and treatment is the worldwide view and attitude toward mental health. The attitude and stigma on mental health treatment and access are major barriers for politicians and policymakers to implement new mental health treatment interventions. The data are clear, comprehensive, and reliable—a positive change in attitude toward mental health treatment would make a significant difference in many life variables worldwide. The change in attitude impacts the availability of treatment, prevention, and promotion of mental health. Treatment for mental health, as evidenced by the data, is as important as physical health. In more developed countries the groups being most overlooked are those with anxiety and depression disorders as well as children with behavioral disorders. Left without treatment, these conditions will develop further and lead to greater levels of disability and societal issues than is necessary. Even more concerning is that those with the most severe mental health conditions are largely untreated in poorer regions of the world (Helliwell et al., 2015; Layard & Hagell, 2015).

Some ways to further address these concerns are by training primary healthcare providers to be much better able to identify and treat mental illness. More than this, a new and larger group of mental health therapists may need to be created with accessibility at the same level as other medical services and community health workers. The greatest overall barrier to effective mental health treatment is in many ways worldwide stigma and beliefs about mental illness. This attitude and collective denial or suppression of the issue only worsens, not helps to resolve, the many ways that mental illness damages individuals and society as a whole. The World Health Assembly adopted a comprehensive mental health action plan to signify a political commitment for countries worldwide to improve mental health (Helliwell et al., 2015; Layard & Hagell, 2015).

LIST OF KEY TAKEAWAYS

- At least 1 in 10 people suffer from mental illness at any time worldwide.
- Depression is the leading cause of disability worldwide, and anxiety is the 6th greatest cause of disability in the world.
- More women than men suffer from both anxiety and depression worldwide. This may in part be due to gender inequality norms that lessen women's power and position.
- Suicide and suicidal ideation related to depression are serious worldwide concerns. According to WHO, over 800,000 people committed suicide in 2017. This is likely an underestimation of actual numbers and does not account for suicidal ideation and attempted suicides.

- There is a significant treatment gap worldwide between mental health needs and actual services provided. Innovative, widespread programs such as Improving Access to Psychological Therapies (IAPT) in the United Kingdom have been significant for understanding the positive impact that easily accessible mental health programs can make on a population-wide basis.

- A majority of mental illness concerns begin in adolescence. A focus on prevention and effective interventions that are easily and regularly accessible is important for addressing these concerns.

REVIEW QUESTIONS

Directions: Refer to what you learned in this chapter as you respond to the questions and prompts below.

1. Define the following terms in your own words in 1 to 2 sentences.

   Happiness
   Depressi
   Purpose
   Mindfulness
   Connection
   Mental Health

2. In 3 to 4 sentences, can you summarize an innovative mental health approach that the British government has implemented?

3. Compare and contrast the general state of mental health between men and women in 1 to 2 sentences.

4. Compare and contrast the general differences between mental health issues and treatment in high-, medium-, and low-income countries in 3 to 4 sentences.

5. What surprised you about this chapter, or what is one thing you learned that you didn't expect beforehand?

REFERENCES

Anālayo, B. (2019). Adding historical depth to definitions of mindfulness. *Current opinion in psychology, 28,* 11–14. https://doi.org/10.1016/j.copsyc.2018.09.013

Baumeister, R., Vohs, K. D., Aaker, J. L., & Gabinsky, E. N. (2013). Some key differences between a happy life and a meaningful life. *The Journal of Positive Psychology, 8,* 505–516. http://dx.doi.org/10.1080/17439760.2013.830764

Bernard, J. E. R. (2018). Depression: A review of its definition. *MOJ Addiction Medicine & Therapy, 5,* 6-7. https://doi.org/10.15406/mojamt.2018.05.00082

Biswas, T., Scott, J. G., Munir, K., Renzaho, A. M., Rawal, L. B., Baxter, J., & Mamun, A. A. (2020). Global variation in the prevalence of suicidal ideation, anxiety, and their correlates among adolescents: a population-based study of 82 countries. *EClinicalMedicine, 24,* 100395.

Clark, A., Fleche, S., Layard, R., Powdthavee, N., & Ward, G. (2017). The key determinants of happiness and misery. In J. F Helliwell, H. Huang, & S. Wang (Eds.), *World happiness report,* (pp. *122-143) Sustainable Development Solutions Network. https://s3.amazonaws.com/happiness-report/2017/HR17.pdf*

George, L. S., & Park, C. L. (2013). Are meaning and purpose distinct? An examination of correlates and predictors. *The Journal of Positive Psychology, 8(5),* 365–375. https://doi.org/10.1080/17439760.2013.805801

Helliwell, J. F., Huang, H., & Wang, S. (2017). The social foundations of world happiness. In J. F Helliwell, H. Huang, & S. Wang (Eds.), *World happiness report,* (pp. *8–47) Sustainable Development Solutions Network. https://s3.amazonaws.com/happiness-report/2017/HR17.pdf*

Helliwell, J. F., Layard, R., & Sachs, J. (Eds.) (2015). *World happiness report 2015.* Sustainable Development Solutions Network. https://worldhappiness.report/ed/2015/

Helliwell, J., Layard, R., & Sachs, J. (Eds.) (2018). *World happiness report 2018,* Sustainable Development Solutions Network. https://worldhappiness.report/ed/2018/

Helliwell, J. F., & Wang, S. (2013). World happiness: Trends, explanations, and distribution. In J. Helliwell, R. Layard, & J. Sachs (Eds.), *World happiness report. Sustainable Development Solutions Network. https://worldhappiness.report/ed/2013/*

Kim-Prieto, C., Diener, E., Tamir, M., Scollon, C. N., & Diener, M. (2005). Integrating the diverse definitions of happiness: A time-sequential framework of subjective well-being. *Journal of Happiness Studies, 6,* 261–300. https://doi.org/10.1007/s10902-005-7226-8

Klussman, K., Curtin, N., Langer, J., & Nichols, A. L. (2022). The importance of awareness, acceptance, and alignment with the self: A framework for understanding self-connection. *Europe's Journal of Psychology, 18(1),* 120–130. https://doi.org/10.5964/ejop.3707

Layard, R., Chisholm, D., Patel, V., & Saxena, S. (2013). Mental illness and unhappiness. (Discussion Paper No. 1239) Center for Economic Performance, London School of Economics and Political Science. https://cep.lse.ac.uk/pubs/download/dp1239.pdf

Layard, R., & Hagell, A. (2015). Healthy young minds: Transforming the mental health of children. In J. F. Helliwell, R. Layard, & J. Sachs (Eds.), *World happiness report (pp.* 106–131). Sustainable Development Solutions Network. https://worldhappiness.report/ed/2015/

World Health Organization. (2017). *Depression and other common mental health disorders: Global health estimates.* World Health Organization. https://apps.who.int/iris/handle/10665/254610

World Health Organization. (2021). *Mental health atlas 2020.* https://www.who.int/publications/i/item/9789240036703

OVERVIEW AND BACKGROUND ON TREATMENT OF MENTAL HEALTH

"The world of the happy is quite another than that of the unhappy."
—Ludwig Wittgenstein

INTRODUCTION

This chapter discusses the evolving and current issues and treatment for mental health in the world and cultural issues that have both positively and negatively impacted the implementation of mental health support and treatment. It provides an overview of major concepts within global mental health treatment and how these concepts can be further applied in the treatment of mental illness. The major concepts covered in this chapter include mental health stigma, mental health literacy, mental health first aid, solution-focused therapy, cognitive behavior therapy, rational emotive behavior therapy, group therapy, yoga and alternative treatment, and family therapy.

KEY TERMS AND DEFINITIONS

Below are common definitions and key terms that will be addressed and used throughout this book and chapter.

Mental Health Stigma

- A significant impediment to effective mental health treatment is cultural and widespread mental health stigma.
- There is greater knowledge about mental illness; however, acceptance of mental illness still ranks towards the bottom of public acceptance.
- Stigma is hypothesized to be as harmful for individuals and society as the experience of untreated mental illness itself. It plays a harmful role, has an effect on an individual's decision to seek treatment, and on underreporting mental illness (Bharadwaj et al., 2017).

Mental Health Literacy

- Mental health literacy (MHL) refers to knowledge about mental health disorders and its understanding, management, and prevention.
- Mental health literacy is another important component of mental health and well-being treatment worldwide (Furnham & Swami, 2018).

- According to Jorm et al. (2010), "mental health literacy" refers to "knowledge and beliefs about mental disorders which aid their recognition, management or prevention" (p.1)

Evidence-Based Therapy

- Evidence-based therapy is supported by research that uses the scientific method and has demonstrated reliable efficacy.
- Acceptance commitment therapy, cognitive behavior therapy, and rational emotive behavior therapy are all evidence-based approaches with the greater potential for worldwide application through psychoeducation, group therapy, government-supported interventions, and clinical therapeutic practice (DiGiuseppe & David, 2015).

Mental Health First Aid

- Mental health first aid training is a method to teach others ways to provide early help for someone who is developing a mental health problem or in a crisis state.
- Mental health first aid training can be provided through e-learning to educate participants on information about mental disorders, stigmatizing attitudes, and helping behaviors.

Overview of Treatment of Mental Health

As you read the section below, please consider the major concepts.

- Mental health stigma and mental health illiteracy are significant impediments to the treatment of mental health disorders worldwide.
- Rational emotive behavior therapy, cognitive behavior therapy, and acceptance and commitment therapy are effective and evidence-based interventions applicable to many populations and situations worldwide.
- Group therapy and complementary and alternative therapy approaches, such as yoga, are significant to consider for global mental health treatment in many regions of the world.

MENTAL HEALTH STIGMA

A significant impediment to effective mental health treatment is cultural and widespread mental health stigma (MHS). Many aspects of human behavior are impacted by the fear of being socially sanctioned or stigmatized. Stigma does not necessarily lead to behavior change but often leads to hiding certain behaviors and actions. Stigma can create a sense of personal shame or negative identity as a result of feeling that a person is deviating from social norms. Stigma has an important negative impact on mental health. There is greater knowledge about mental illness; however, acceptance of mental illness still ranks towards the bottom of public acceptance. Stigma is serious as it prevents and deters individuals from seeking mental health care. Stigma is hypothesized to be as harmful to individuals and society as the experience of untreated mental illness itself. It plays a harmful role, has an effect on an individual's decision to seek treatment, and on underreporting mental illness (Bharadwaj et al., 2017).

MHS is also significant in terms of the financial impact that untreated and pervasive mental illness has on society. It is predicted that the cost of mental illness is between US$60 billion to $300 billion annually in the United States alone. Aside from this, MHS and the associated lack of treatment lead to decreased self-esteem and self-efficacy. This impacts job productivity, unemployment, and job functioning. Individuals with mental illness are much more likely to be unemployed and underemployed than individuals without mental illness. In addition to this, at least 30% of individuals with severe mental illness encounter discrimination in both trying to obtain or maintain employment. Other forms of stigma associated with MHS include friend stigma, health insurance stigma, housing stigma, and family stigma. Early and consistent mental health treatment has positive outcomes for individuals, families, and society as a whole (Sickel et al., 2014).

A compounding factor with MHS is the issue of toxic masculinity. Conventional ideas about masculinity create a worsening of MHS. Masculine norms are strongly associated with the underuse of the health system, including mental health services. Traditional masculine norms and toxic masculinity are both modes of thinking and operating that lead to difficulty expressing emotions, identifying mental health needs, and seeking services. These norms lead to worsening depression, anxiety, substance abuse, health risks, interpersonal relationship concerns, increased violence, worsening psychological distress, and reduced motivation to seek help. Redefining masculinity and manhood are key components to combat this toxic masculinity and the negative impacts it has. It is important that men are able to express themselves and seek help for mental illness symptoms (Chatmon, 2020).

Mental illness is an issue that negatively impacts the well-being of an unknown number of individuals worldwide. However, despite the high prevalence levels of mental illness, a large number of individuals who need treatment do not receive it. MHS is a major impediment to finding and obtaining mental health treatment. It impacts all life components and significantly influences numerous overall health outcomes. The mental health issue of greatest global concern is major depression, and close to 50% of U.S. adults experience a mental illness during their lifetime. Treating MHS is an important consideration for effective interventions regarding mental illness (Sickel et al., 2014).

MENTAL HEALTH LITERACY

Mental health literacy (MHL) refers to knowledge about mental health disorders and their understanding, management, and prevention. MHL is another important component of mental health and well-being treatment worldwide (Furnham & Swami, 2018). According to Jorm et al. (2010), "mental health literacy" refers to "knowledge and beliefs about mental disorders which aid their recognition, management or prevention" (p.1) It consists of (a) the ability to recognize mental health disorders and mental distress, (b) understanding and knowledge of causes and risk factors, (c) information and understanding of self-help interventions, (d) information and understanding of available professional assistance, (e) understanding about help-seeking, and (f) knowledge of how to seek and obtain mental health information and treatment (Jorm, 2010). If MHL is not improved, it will likely continue to hinder the public's acceptance of evidence-based mental health care and interfere with treatment, self-help, and community support of mental illness concerns. Health literacy is defined as "the ability to gain access to, understand, and use information in ways which promote and maintain good health" (Furnham & Swami, 2018) The importance of health literacy for physical health is widely accepted; however, there is a lack of acknowledgment of the importance of mental health literacy (Furnham & Swami, 2018).

Research has demonstrated that the general public has a poor understanding of mental illness symptoms and is more accepting of self-help approaches over traditional medical treatment. Variables such as age, gender, education, culture, and urban versus rural living differences are relevant for variations in mental health literacy. However, in spite of this, two of the United Nations' sustainable development goals include good health and well-being. According to the World Health Organization, health literacy is a stronger predictor of health than factors such as education, income, employment, and ethnic group. WHO estimates that at least one-third of the population worldwide suffers from a mental illness, with the most common conditions being anxiety, depression, and mood disorders. The high rates of mental illness worldwide create many consequences for societies and families, and a majority with mental illness do not receive any professional treatment (Furnham & Swami, 2018).

MHL in developing countries is poorly understood and misunderstood. The training of primary health care professionals on MHL is a critical component to improve the treatment of populations in need, particularly in low- and middle-income countries where mental health services are limited. Efforts to increase MHL in low- and middle-income countries need to be innovative and inclusive. Existing resources in developed and developing countries need to be effectively used to improve mental health services and access to treatment. Indicators such as number of psychiatrists per population, availability of psychotropic medications, and integration level of mental health services into primary care are all important components of inadequate mental health care. Other important mechanisms to improve mental health literacy include awareness campaigns, educational workshops, training courses, and mental health first aid training (Ganasen et al., 2008).

Mental disorders often appear visibly for the first time in adolescence and with young adults. Early recognition and treatment are critical for better long-term outcomes. However, the evidence shows that professional treatment is not obtained or even sought until after the symptoms have been pervasive for a period of time. Early intervention will most likely only occur if children and their caregivers can identify early signs and indications of mental illness and how to access help. Four types of interventions can work to improve mental health literacy, these include (a) whole-of-community campaigns, (b) youth audience community campaigns,

(c) school-based interventions teaching help-seeking skills, mental health literacy, and resilience, and (d) and programs training others to better intervene in a mental health crisis. Health promotion models can be effective for improving general mental health literacy. This is important for prevention and early intervention for youth struggling with mental illness (Kelly et al., 2007).

A majority of the public cannot recognize specific mental health disorders or understand psychological distress. In general, the public differs from mental health experts in their understanding and beliefs about mental disorders and effective treatments. Attitudes that interfere with identification and help-seeking behavior are pervasive. MHL to the general public can be greatly improved as a majority of existing mental health information available to the public is incorrect. This issue should be adequately addressed as an important factor for well-being, happiness, and mental health intervention in every region of the world (Jorm, 2000).

MENTAL HEALTH FIRST AID

Mental health first aid training (MHFA) is a method to teach others ways to provide early help for someone who is developing a mental health problem or in a crisis state. MHFA training can be provided through e-learning to educate participants on information about mental disorders, stigmatizing attitudes, and helping behaviors. MHFA training has been shown through both e-learning and printed manual materials, to increase knowledge, reduce stigma, and improve self-confidence. Also, e-learning can be more effective than printed manual learning materials for reducing stigma and disability from mental illness. Training trainers on mental health first aid is also an effective way to increase the use, dissemination, and application of the information, as well as improve mental health literacy (Jorm et al., 2010).

MHFA consists of five steps. The first step is to assess the risk of suicide or harm of an individual. The second step is to listen nonjudgmentally to the individual seeking support. The third step is to provide reassurance and information to the distressed person or group. The fourth step is to provide encouragement to the distressed person/group and to obtain appropriate professional assistance. The fifth step is to encourage self-help strategies for the distressed individual/group (Kitchener & Jorm, 2006). Research has demonstrated that through MHFA training, a whole community can provide aid through formal mental health services with early identification and intervention of mental illness (Kitchener & Jorm, 2008).

SOLUTION-FOCUSED THERAPY

Solution-focused therapy focuses on the strengths individuals already possess and the belief that people already have the resources they need to solve their own problems. A growing body of evidence offers support for this therapy approach, and many applications can be potentially incorporated into mental health literacy literature and mental health first aid interventions (Corcoran & Pillai, 2009). Solution-focused brief therapy (SFBT) is a future-focused, goal-oriented brief therapy. Insoo Kim Berg, Steve de Shazer, and colleagues at the Milwaukee Brief Family Therapy Center created SFBT at the beginning of the 1980s. They developed it by observing hundreds of hours of therapy over the years and noting the questions, behaviors, and emotions that helped clients figure out solutions and enact improvements in their lives. SFBT is developed from pragmatic observations, an approach that focuses on identifying what is working in relationships and situations, and building on what is working. An important distinction of SFBT is its focus and language on solutions, not on problems (De Shazer et al., 2021).

The language of problems is different from the language and perspective of solutions. Some central components of SFBT are that:

1) If something works, do more of it
2) If something is not broken, don't change it
3) If it's not working, do something different
4) (Small steps can result in big changes
5) Solutions are not necessarily directly related to the problem
6) Look for exceptions in the problem; no problems happen all the time
7) The future is not known; it is created and flexible.

Solution-focused therapy is a highly successful, popular, and extensively used therapy in the world. It is grounded in pragmatism, resiliency, the client's own history of solutions, and exceptions to the problems; it can be applied to all problems. SFBT works to build on an individual's strengths and resiliencies; it helps them identify these aspects and increase those behaviors (De Shazer et al., 2021).

COGNITIVE BEHAVIOR THERAPY

Cognitive behavioral therapy (CBT) is a well-known and widely used therapeutic approach, both through psychoeducation and traditional therapy for numerous problems globally. In an investigation of 269 meta-analysis studies, the application of CBT was found to positively impact symptoms from the following conditions: substance use disorders, schizophrenia and other types of psychosis, depression, mood disorder, anxiety disorder, bipolar disorder, eating disorder, insomnia, personality disorder, anger, criminal behavior, stress, chronic pain and fatigue, distress related to medical conditions, and more. From this investigation, CBT demonstrated the best results in treating anxiety, bulimia, anger, stress, and somatoform disorders. CBT is a very strong evidence-based approach. It is used worldwide and supported by many government-sponsored mental health initiatives such as in the United Kingdom (Hofmann et al., 2012).

CBT has been integrated into even more effective, evidence-based approaches with the growth of mindfulness-based treatments and acceptance and commitment therapy (ACT). These approaches have a basis in CBT but also deviate from traditional CBT practices. Deviations in CBT provide a foundation to create a greater base of intervention and treatment for psychoeducation and population-wide interventions. CBT may best be understood as a family of interventions that can be adapted to treat numerous emotional disorders. Mindfulness-based cognitive therapy is one such approach that both integrates CBT and also deviates from its norms. Mindfulness-based treatments focus on a present-moment, nonjudgmental approach. Mindfulness interventions help bring awareness and insight into problematic and harmful thought patterns so that they can be reconsidered and reframed in a new, positive manner. Dialectical behavior therapy (DBT) is another offshoot of CBT that combines structured mindfulness-based techniques with acceptance and change as a central component of emotional regulation. DBT emphasizes acceptance, emotional distress tolerance, and insight into cognitions, emotions, and behaviors (Hofmann et al., 2010).

A way to increasingly implement these differing effective and evidence-based approaches is e-mental health. E-mental health refers to mental health services and information delivered or enhanced through the internet and related technology. It is a viable option for individuals without access to traditional face-to-face therapy. Important components of CBT with e-mental health include cognitive restructuring, behavior change, exposure, and problem-solving. E-mental health is of growing use and interest to address mental health needs and conditions in recent years. Mobile health apps are effective for mental health interventions alongside CBT. CBT techniques can be effectively applied to mental health apps, to support self-help as well as psychoeducational needs, and address larger numbers of individuals. E-mental health is also an effective way to provide support and a kind of treatment for individuals with mental disorders and limited resources. (Denecke et al., 2022).

RATIONAL EMOTIVE BEHAVIOR THERAPY

Rational emotive behavior therapy (REBT) was created by Albert Ellis in the 1950s and is considered the baseline and original cognitive behavior therapy. REBT has been reviewed in clinical and nonclinical populations, children, adolescents, adults, educational, military, and business settings. It has been studied among many populations and groupings. Ellis's and Beck's works are foundational components of CBT. The main focus of REBT is irrational and rational beliefs. CBT is more focused on automatic thinking and schema. Hayes's acceptance and commitment therapy is related to these but focuses on reactions to thoughts, emotions, and images instead of reframing and cognitive restructuring. REBT helps individuals to change irrational beliefs to rational beliefs and thereby better cope with reality and any difficult circumstances. ACT, CBT, and REBT are all evidence-based approaches with greater application worldwide through psychoeducation, group therapy, government-supported interventions, and clinical therapeutic practice (DiGiuseppe & David, 2015).

Important components of REBT are the understanding that rigidity is a central core aspect of psychological disturbance, and flexibility is the core of psychological health. This rigidity is expressed through an individual's belief systems. Specifically, rigid beliefs lead to extreme beliefs, and flexible beliefs lead to nonextreme beliefs. REBT and CBT challenge the thoughts that create a disturbance. REBT is psychoeducational because it posits that individuals can be taught skills to identify, challenge, and replace their dysfunctional beliefs on their own. It provides a good opportunity for larger, global mental health workers because of this psychoeducational component and aspect that increases resiliency through fostering greater flexibility and non-extreme belief structures. Critical components of REBT that are supportive for populations in various populations include self-acceptance, nonutopian, high-frustration tolerance, self-responsibility for disturbance, acceptance of uncertainty, commitment to something outside of yourself, flexibility in thinking, and self-responsibility for disturbance instead of blaming others. It involves finding in what areas a person can empower themselves and being accountable for negative beliefs and negative reactions to those beliefs (Jordana et al., 2020).

GROUP SUPPORT AND GROUP THERAPY

Group counseling provides a method to deliver information, impact larger numbers of people, and help an individual counselor have more time for a greater number of clients. Group therapy, group support, and group psychoeducation are effective for helping individuals in group experiences to learn skills to function effectively, foster distress tolerance and manage negative emotions with stress and anxiety, and to develop better skills for working and living with others. Group counseling provides an innovative outlet for giving support to greater numbers of people (Berg et al., 2017).

Group counseling can also be used preventatively as a way to teach individuals skills to manage negative emotions and challenges and increase positive emotions. This can include education on how to do self-help mechanisms such as REBT, mindfulness interventions, self-compassion, and other teachable tools. Preventive group psychoeducational therapy can be a useful approach to help individuals and also potentially bypass the concerns regarding mental health literacy and mental health stigma. Groups are taught preventative measures and skills to improve their mental health if they are struggling or if they struggle in the future. It also provides education on mental health and well-being to address cultural misconceptions and misunderstandings (Berg et al., 2017).

Group support can also be provided through 12-step interventions and peer support. Peer-led groups have been found to be effective ways to increase support and psychoeducation for individuals struggling with a variety of concerns. It can also be a way to address mental health literacy and some mental health stigma through anonymous, peer-led support. Twelve-step mutual support programs are easily available either remotely online or in person, and represent no cost to community-based resources for these individuals. Twelve-step groups are useful for substance abuse addictions, food addictions, gambling, sex addictions, codependency concerns, and other potentially unidentified applications that have yet to be used. The 12-step philosophy looks at a certain view and perspective in the recovery process. It considers addiction as a kind of disease and works to increase individual maturity and spiritual growth, decrease self-centeredness, and provide help to others suffering from addiction. The first step in this 12-step process is admitting that one has an issue with addiction. This type of curriculum-based, structured peer-led support group offers anonymous support, can provide psychoeducation, and be a good alternative for resource-poor areas with poor mental health literacy (Donovan et al., 2013).

YOGA

Yoga is an increasingly important complementary and alternative medical treatment for mental health disorders. Complementary and alternative medicine can be effective in providing mental health support in areas of mental health stigma, mental health illiteracy, and resource-poor regions in which paying for mental health services is not viable. Yoga is considered a type of complementary and alternative medical treatment and has been used for thousands of years for good physical and mental health. Yoga can be applied for prevention, health promotion, and also for the support of mental health disorders (Gangadhar & Varambally, 2011).

FAMILY THERAPY

Family therapy is a term for working with families with biopsychosocial challenges. Family therapy looks at relational difficulties among family members and also systems. This approach can be helpful for promoting mental health literacy and reducing stigma. Family therapy and systems therapy is a growing approach that goes beyond traditional individual therapeutic practices. It can be worthwhile to consider future applications of this modality in other cultures and how it can be used in a larger way (Carr, 2012).

LIST OF KEY TAKEAWAYS

- Mental health stigma and mental health illiteracy are major barriers worldwide to effective interventions regarding well-being, happiness, and mental health.
- Approaches such as CBT, REBT, DBT, ACT, and solution-focused therapy are evidence-based, effective approaches that can be used with many different population groups worldwide.
- Group therapy and alternative approaches such as yoga, e-mental health, and systems-based interventions can be effective ways to provide some kind of treatment.
- Psychoeducation and e-mental health are growing in relevancy as methods to provide greater prevention, education, and treatment.

REVIEW QUESTIONS

Directions: Refer to what you learned in this chapter to respond to the questions and prompts below.

- In 3 to 4 sentences, summarize a potentially effective approach that can generally increase mental health care.
- How is mental health stigma harmful to mental health treatment?
- What is the potential harm of mental health illiteracy?
- What surprised you about this chapter, or what is one thing you learned that you didn't expect?

REFERENCES

Berg, R. C., Landreth, G. L., & Fall, K. A. (2017). *Group counseling: Concepts and procedures*. Routledge.

Bharadwaj, P., Pai, M. M., & Suziedelyte, A. (2017). Mental health stigma. *Economics Letters*, *159*, 57–60. https://doi.org/10.1016/j.econlet.2017.06.028

Carr, A. (2012). *Family therapy: Concepts, process and practice*. John Wiley & Sons.

Chatmon, B. N. (2020). Males and mental health stigma. *American Journal of Men's Health*, *14*(4). https://doi.org/10.1177/1557988320949322

Corcoran, J., & Pillai, V. (2009). A review of the research on solution-focused therapy. *British Journal of Social Work*, *39*(2), 234–242. https://doi.org/10.1093/bjsw/bcm098

Denecke, K., Schmid, N., & Nüssli, S. (2022). Implementation of cognitive behavioral therapy in e–mental health apps: Literature review. *Journal of Medical Internet Research*, *24*(3), e27791. https://doi.org/10.2196/27791

De Shazer, S., Dolan, Y., Korman, H., Trepper, T., McCollum, E., & Berg, I. K. (2021). *More than miracles: The state of the art of solution-focused brief therapy*. Routledge.

DiGiuseppe, R., & David, O. A. (2015). Rational emotive behavior therapy. In H. T. Prout & A. L. Fedewa (Eds.), *Counseling and psychotherapy with children and adolescents: Theory and practice for school and clinical settings* (pp. 155–215). John Wiley & Sons Inc.

Donovan, D. M., Ingalsbe, M. H., Benbow, J., & Daley, D. C. (2013). 12-step interventions and mutual support programs for substance use disorders: An overview. *Social Work in Public Health*, *28*(3–4),313–332. https://doi.org/

Furnham, A., & Swami, V. (2018). Mental health literacy: A review of what it is and why it matters. *International Perspectives in Psychology: Research, Practice, Consultation*, *7*(4), 240–257. https://doi.org/10.1037/ipp0000094

Ganasen, K. A., Parker, S., Hugo, C. J., Stein, D. J., Emsley, R. A., & Seedat, S. (2008). Mental health literacy: Focus on developing countries. *African Journal of Psychiatry*, *11*(1), 23–28. https://doi.org/10.4314/ajpsy.v11i1.30251

Gangadhar, B. N., & Varambally, S. (2011). Yoga as therapy in psychiatric disorders: Past, present, and future. *Biofeedback*, *39*(2), 60–63. https://doi.org/10.5298/1081-5937-39.2.03

Hofmann, S. G., Asnaani, A., Vonk, I. J., Sawyer, A. T., & Fang, A. (2012). The efficacy of cognitive behavioral therapy: A review of meta-analyses. *Cognitive Therapy and Research*, *36*, 427–440. https://doi.org/10.1007/s10608-012-9476-1

Hofmann, S. G., Sawyer, A. T., & Fang, A. (2010). The empirical status of the "new wave" of cognitive behavioral therapy. *Psychiatric Clinics*, *33*(3), 701–710. https://doi.org/10.1016/j.psc.2010.04.006

Jordana, A., Turner, M. J., Ramis, Y., & Torregrossa, M. (2020). A systematic mapping review on the use of rational emotive behavior therapy (REBT) with athletes. *International Review of Sport and Exercise Psychology*, 1–26. https://doi.org/10.1080/1750984X.2020.1836673

Jorm, A. F. (2000). Mental health literacy: Public knowledge and beliefs about mental disorders. *The British Journal of Psychiatry*, *177*(5), 396–401. https://doi.org/10.1192/bjp.177.5.396

Jorm, A. F., Kitchener, B. A., Fischer, J. A., & Cvetkovski, S. (2010). Mental health first aid training by e-learning: A randomized controlled trial. *Australian & New Zealand Journal of Psychiatry*, *44*(12),1072–1081. https://doi.org/10.3109/00048674.2010.516426

Kelly, C. M., Jorm, A. F., & Wright, A. (2007). Improving mental health literacy as a strategy to facilitate early intervention for mental disorders. *Medical Journal of Australia*, *187*(S7), S26–S30. https://doi.org/10.5694/j.1326-5377.2007.tb01332.x

Kitchener, B. A., & Jorm, A. F. (2006). Mental health first aid training: Review of evaluation studies. *Australian & New Zealand Journal of Psychiatry*, *40*(1), 6–8. https://doi.org/10.1080/j.1440-1614.2006.01735.x

Kitchener, B. A., & Jorm, A. F. (2008). Mental health first aid: An international programme for early intervention. *Early Intervention in Psychiatry*, *2*(1), 55–61. https://doi.org/10.1111/j.1751-7893.2007.00056.x

Sickel, A. E., Seacat, J. D., & Nabors, N. A. (2014). Mental health stigma update: A review of consequences. *Advances in Mental Health*, *12*(3), 202–215. https://doi.org/10.1080/18374905.2014.11081898

MENTAL HEALTH, TREATMENT, AND HAPPINESS IN LATIN AMERICA

"I have a wonderful shelter, which is my family."
—Jose Carreras

INTRODUCTION

Latin America reports high levels of happiness in spite of high levels of crime, mental illness, and poverty. This region demonstrates unexpectedly and paradoxically high levels of subjective well-being, happiness, and mental health in comparison to other parts of the world and from what would be predicted by income levels and the relationship to income and well-being. The Latin American region is comprised of Brazil and 18 Spanish-speaking countries including Argentina, Bolivia, Chile, Colombia, Costa Rica, Cuba, Dominican Republic, Ecuador, El Salvador, Guatemala, Honduras, Mexico, Nicaragua, Panama, Paraguay, Peru, Uruguay, and Venezuela. Puerto Rico is another region with many Latin American influences. Haiti is part of the region but has a different history and culture from the Spanish- and Portuguese-speaking countries in the surrounding region. As of 2018, this region had a population of about 620 million people, and no country in this region was considered high-income based on per capita income. This region is full of diversity, but there is a general sense of an overall culture throughout the area (Graham & Nikolova, 2018; Helliwell et al., 2018; Rojas, 2018).

KEY TERMS AND DEFINITIONS

Below are common definitions and key terms that will be addressed and used throughout this book and chapter.

Latin America

- Latin America refers to the region of the world consisting of the entire continent of South America as well as Mexico, Central America, and the Caribbean islands using Romance-language dialects.
- This region experienced conquest by the Spaniards and Portuguese from the late 15*th* through the 18*th* century.
- This region consists of great variations in cultures, geography, and climate. It is connected through the history and influence of the Spaniards and Portuguese in its history (Graham & Nikolova, 2018; Helliwell et al., 2018; Rojas, 2018).

The Caracas Declaration

- A milestone event was the Regional Conference for the Restructuring of Psychiatric Care in Latin America in Caracas, Venezuela, in 1990.
- A result of this conference was the Caracas Declaration, which created a set of principles to serve as a conceptual framework for the reform work that would occur in later years.
- This conference created a commitment to transform outdated hospital-based mental health systems into comprehensive community care (Minoletti et al., 2012).

Crime Victimization

- Crime victimization is a significant objective issue and factor in Latin American life satisfaction and happiness.
- According to the Barometer Survey of 2014, the public opinion poll in Latin America that collects self-reported measures of life satisfaction, the greatest impediment to positive mental health and happiness in Latin America is crime victimization.
- Latin America has the second highest rate of crime victimization in the world (Ortega Londoño et al., 2019).

Underrepresented Groups in Latin America

- Underrepresented groups generally experience worse levels of mental health in Latin America.
- These groups include LGBTQ, indigenous populations, rural low-income populations, and criminal offenders (Almanzar et al., 2015).
- Other groups that experience high risk and levels of mental illness are women, children, and the elderly (Nepomuceno et al., 2016).

The Latin American Paradox

- The Latin American paradox refers to the uncharacteristically high levels of happiness and well-being in Latin America with its accompanying high levels of poverty.
- This is sometimes also referred to as the happiness paradox. In contrast, the Easterlin Paradox indicates that happiness and economic prosperity are strongly associated to a certain degree.
- However, the Latin American paradox provides contradictory data with uncharacteristically high happiness levels and low economic prosperity (Graham & Nikolova, 2018; Helliwell et al., 2018; Rojas, 2018).

Overview and Background of Mental Health in Latin America

As you read the section below, please consider the paradox and unique circumstances in Latin America and how mental health and happiness are important cultural and societal concerns of the region.

- Latin America has one of the highest rates of homicide and criminal victimization in the world.
- The high levels of criminal victimization have significant negative mental health and well-being impacts on survivors.
- Latin American countries consistently rank in the top tiers for happiness worldwide in spite of the high levels of societal violence.
- Latin America suffers from high rates of mental illness.
- Lifetime mental health disorder prevalence in Latin America ranges from 23.7% to 39.1%.
- Twelve-month prevalence of mental illness in the region ranges from 11.6% to 20.1%.
- It is estimated that mental health disorders make up about 20% of total disease burden in Latin America.
- The high mental illness and high levels of crime victimization create a paradox with its accompanying high levels of happiness

---

HISTORY OF LATIN AMERICAN REGION AND WELL-BEING

Research on mental health, subjective well-being, and happiness has identified that Latin America is a region with high life evaluation indicators in contrast to income level. Positive affect is outstandingly high compared to the rest of the world. The history of the Spanish and Europeans in this region is different from other parts of the world where colonization took place. The large indigenous populations were not eradicated or segregated. The Europeans and indigenous groups mixed and created *mestizo,* which is a mix of European and indigenous ancestry. Latin American culture has evolved over the last 500 years during European colonial rule and 200 years of independence. During this 500-year period, the values and perspectives of the indigenous people have merged with that of the Spanish and Portuguese population. In many ways, it is a history of coexistence and blending between the European and indigenous groups (Graham & Nikolova, 2018; Helliwell et al., 2018; Rojas, 2018).

The blend of these two cultures led to a society that emphasized connection and interpersonal relations between family and relatives. The combination of native indigenous, Spanish and Portuguese values led to a society that appreciated and embraced family ties, extended family and warm, close and enjoyable relationships. Overall, the Latin American culture values relationships with others as a focal point and central part of one's life purpose (Graham & Nikolova, 2018; Helliwell et al., 2018; Rojas, 2018).

Therefore, the family is a very important part of positive emotional development and purpose. In Latin America, people generally live with their families longer than in other parts of the world and do not necessarily leave their families as adults. This is in contrast to many common western ideas that once someone is an adult they should move out and leave the home. As a result of living with their family longer, they tend to develop deeper relationships with those they grow up with and have long-lasting relationships. It is estimated that approximately one-third of adults still live with their parents in contrast to 12% in Western Europe and 9% in Anglo-Saxon countries (Graham & Nikolova, 2018; Helliwell et al., 2018; Rojas, 2018).

As a result of the unique nature and dynamic of well-being and happiness in the Latin America region it is important to look at subjective well-being. Other regions emphasize and find greater understanding through measurements of objective variables such as income, health, and education levels. Subjective well-being helps us consider cultural values and understand intention and behavior. The Latin America data are important as they highlight otherwise overlooked variables for well-being, specifically concerning subjective, positive relational variables (Graham & Nikolova, 2018; Helliwell et al., 2018; Rojas, 2018).

LATIN AMERICA AND HAPPINESS

The positive affective state is particularly high in Latin American countries. They generally rank in the upper levels for well-being and happiness despite not being at the highest levels of income and other wealth factors such as education and employment. The research on Latin America highlights the importance of accounting for the affective state when assessing happiness. Latin American countries range from an average of 7.15 in Costa Rica to 4.93 in the Dominican Republic. The average ranking, according to the 2018 Gallup World Poll, is 6.07 on an estimated scale of 1-10 on the Life Evaluation Index where scores of 4 or less represent suffering, scores of 5-6 represent struggling, and scores of 7+ represent thriving. Latin American levels of happiness are much higher than the average ranking in the world at 5.42. A unique case study within Latin America is Costa Rica with its very unusually high ranking of well-being at 7.15 (Graham & Nikolova, 2018; Helliwell et al., 2018; Rojas, 2018). Some factors that help explain the unique situation in Costa Rica include the relatively good welfare system in the country, which provides universal health care, and primary and secondary education. Also, Costa Rica has had no army since 1949. Costa Rica's level of well-being ranks higher than the average Western European country (Graham & Nikolova, 2018; Helliwell et al., 2018; Rojas, 2018).

From 2006 to 2016, eight of the top 10 countries worldwide are Latin American, and 10 out of the top 15 countries in the world for positive affect are Latin American. In addition to this, the negative effect in this region of the world is not low, which adds to its higher overall rankings. Some countries such as Bolivia, Peru, and Venezuela stand out as having higher levels of negative affect due to economic crisis, political polarization, high levels of violence, and family instability due to migration and immigration. However, overall, the data from Latin America demonstrate a high positive effect when compared to corresponding income, which is in contradiction to most explanatory variables for well-being. Therefore, Latin American countries on the whole are outliers to what "should be" their levels of happiness when using common explanatory factors. The data reflect that social organization provides a buffer to economic concerns and encourages and promotes increased happiness levels overall (Graham & Nikolova, 2018; Helliwell et al., 2018; Rojas, 2018;).

THE ANOMALY OF LATIN AMERICAN WELL-BEING

One significant factor in the differentiation of Latin America in happiness and well-being is its focus on additional aspects of importance other than income. In Latin America, per capita incomes are not low, and there is a reasonable availability of public goods, health, and education services in a majority of the countries. Numerous Latin American countries are categorized by the United Nations Development Programme as "high human development." Also, the high happiness levels in Latin America are not seen as an abnormality or anomaly in the culture. It is understood to be related to the abundance of family warmth and a wealth of supportive social relationships (Graham & Nikolova, 2018; Helliwell et al., 2018; Rojas, 2018). This is directly in line with the most recent well-being research that points to the connection between relationships and individual happiness. The better and more abundant our relationships, the greater our levels of happiness. Latin America in general has strong social foundations and an abundance of positive relationships. This is a unique finding when comparing this region to the rest of the world and particularly to areas such as the United States (Graham & Nikolova, 2018; Helliwell et al., 2018; Rojas, 2018).

The abundant social relationships in Latin America provide a buffer and protection against life satisfaction problems that can be related to the levels of corruption, violence, crime, and economic difficulties. A point of interest is that these patterns of interpersonal relations are different from other patterns of interpersonal relations otherwise seen throughout the world. There is a greater sense of purpose through relationships, or, rather, a relational purpose is associated with higher levels of happiness (Graham & Nikolova, 2018; Helliwell et al., 2018; Rojas, 2018).

LATIN AMERICA AND MENTAL ILLNESS

On the whole, Latin America has a significant prevalence of mental illness. Community-based epidemiological studies in the Latin America region estimate rates of lifetime mental health disorder prevalence range from 23.7% to 39.1%, and 12-month prevalence ranges from 11.6% to 20.1%. It is estimated that mental health disorders make up about 20% of total disease burden in Latin America (Minoletti et al., 2012). During the 1950s and 1960s, epidemiological studies were conducted covering the 20 countries in Latin America. These studies used case studies and random sampling methods to assess the prevalence of mental illness throughout different countries and to question the dominant role of psychiatric hospitals. Within these studies, suggestions and ideas to use alternative models that incorporate general hospitals, primary care, group homes, and outpatient care for individuals with severe mental health disorders were explored. During this time, innovative pilot programs were also attempted that combined efforts with psychiatrists, general practitioners, and other health professionals (Minoletti et al., 2012). These studies in the 1950s and 1960s were early attempts at revolutionizing an antiquated, costly, inflexible mental health system. Unfortunately, due to inadequate political support and resources, this updated community model was never fully implemented. However, it provided a foundation to create change and cultivated awareness and education regarding psychiatric hospital alternatives (Minoletti et al., 2012).

Sara Anne Spowart

MENTAL HEALTH INVESTMENT IN LATIN AMERICA

Mental health disorders are very prevalent in Latin American countries and create a significant negative impact on society, families, and cultures as a whole. However, investment in public mental health is inadequate. Positive improvements have been made during the last 22 years due to leadership and influence from the Pan American Health Organization/World Health Organization (PAHO/WHO). PAHO/WHO worked to create national policies, plans, and local programs to provide specialized community care for individuals with severe mental health conditions. Currently, most Latin American countries have a model of care for severe mental health concerns that is based on psychiatric hospitals. This model does not lend itself to prevention and effective treatment. Also, it is very costly and takes up most of the national mental health budget. Some potential solutions include (a) multi-country studies on community services, (b) an investigation of new approaches and interventions already existing in countries with more advanced mental health services, (c) strengthening advocacy groups through cross-country interchange, and (d) creating a network of well-trained leaders to leapfrog growth throughout the area (Minoletti et al., 2012).

In the 1970s and 1980s, a majority of these innovative programs were downscaled or forced to close as a result of political dictatorships. During this time period of dictatorships, more psychiatric hospitals were built, with over 250 psychiatric hospitals existing and over 150,000 long-stay beds. The treatment at these hospitals was inhumane in many cases, with patients in isolation, physically restrained, and heavily sedated with psychiatric drugs. In multiple countries, psychiatric hospitals like these were the only accessible mental health treatment option. This shifted back again with democracy returning to Latin America in the 1990s. During this time, long-standing mental health issues were able to be addressed. Psychiatrists Benedetto Saraceno of Nicaragua and Franco Basaglia of Brazil, were particularly significant in this era. Basaglia had been involved as a leader in the Italian movement for psychiatric change in the 1970s and 1980s. Their work had an impact in two major ways—specifically, the possibility of transforming asylums into a network of community centers and ensuring patients are citizens with equal rights to other people (Minoletti et al., 2012).

THE CARACAS DECLARATION AND LATIN AMERICAN MENTAL HEALTH

A milestone event was the Regional Conference for the Restructuring of Psychiatric Care in Latin America in Caracas, Venezuela, in 1990. A result of this conference was the Caracas Declaration, which created a set of principles to serve as a conceptual framework for the reform work that would occur in later years. This conference created a commitment to transform outdated hospital-based mental health systems into comprehensive community care. It also focused on the protection of human rights for people with mental health concerns. Another important consideration in the progression of mental health treatment in Latin America includes WHO-AIMS studies that demonstrate low priority to mental health. Other important components of the Caracas agenda include self-care and informal care, mental health in primary care, outpatient treatment for severe mental illness, daycare programs, psychosocial rehabilitation, and incorporation of mental health services in general hospitals. Through this declaration, the first line of care is (1) self-care, followed by (2) informal community care, (3) primary health care services, (4) community mental health, (5) outpatient psychiatry, (6) intensive outpatient care, and (7) lastly hospital care (Minoletti et al., 2012).

However, in spite of the Caracas Declaration, the change and movement away from hospital care has been slow or even nonexistent in some Latin American countries. Only three Latin American countries, Brazil, Chile, and Panama have really moved away from the psychiatric hospital-based model. There has been a reduction in hospital bed usage in other countries, but it is still slow. In other countries in the area there has been only a 23.9% reduction in mental hospital beds in the last 10 years. Brazil, Chile, and Panama have been successful with reducing the use of psychiatric hospital beds by 62.2% in the last 10 years. In addition to this, Brazil and Chile have an increasing number of community group homes for individuals with severe mental illness and inadequate family support. This incredible change in Brazil, Chile, and Panama is a result of significant public mental health expenditures to general hospitals, outpatient facilities, and community services. Belize is another success case within the Latin American region. It has significantly downsized its use of mental hospital beds and provided mental health care training to primary care psychiatric nurses in every health district (Minoletti et al., 2012).

Aside from this, another important consideration is combatting stigma and discrimination that can be associated with mental illness in Latin America. Addressing this stigma and discrimination is a key component of helping individuals utilize and seek out community resources. There have been many great examples of progress since the Caracas Declaration. However, a majority of countries in Latin America still have a psychiatric hospital-care model for mental health treatment. Some factors that hinder enacting reforms include a weak political will to make changes, a low allocation to mental health funding in government budgets, a lack of legislation to protect the human rights of individuals with mental illness, and the continuation of high-cost, inappropriate mental health care (Minoletti et al., 2012).

CRIME VICTIMIZATION IN LATIN AMERICA

A significant objective issue and factor in Latin American life satisfaction and happiness is the concern over crime victimization. According to the Barometer Survey of 2014, the public opinion poll in Latin America that collects self-reported measures of life satisfaction, the greatest impediment to positive mental health and happiness in Latin America is crime victimization (Ortega Londoño et al., 2019). The results of this poll demonstrate the negative relationship between being a victim of crime and individual levels of life satisfaction. This survey also found that the most significant factor in well-being is being a direct victim of crime rather than living in a country with high rates of homicide. The individual or direct experience of crime impacts one's level of well-being. It also has social costs, private costs, and government or public costs. Latin America has the second highest rate of crime victimization in the world; only sub-Saharan Africa is higher (Ortega Londoño et al., 2019).

Growth of Crime in Latin America

Latin America and the Caribbean make up 33% of homicides worldwide, but the region constitutes only 9% of the world's population. This is a major discrepancy and has created a culture of crime. In addition, Latin America is the only region in the world where violence has continually grown since 2005. Reducing crime in the area would positively impact society in numerous different ways and increase life satisfaction, well-being, and happiness. Crime victimization has a significant negative impact on life satisfaction, mental health, and happiness (Ortega Londoño et al., 2019).

Paradox of Crime, Victimization, and Well-Being

However, in spite of the extremely high levels of direct crime victimization, most countries in the Latin America region are ranked in the top 50 happiest countries in the world. This is an unusual paradox not seen in other areas of the globe. Countries with higher levels of criminality also report higher levels of happiness. According to Ortega Londoño et al. (2019), being a victim of a crime in the last year lowers the likelihood of an individual reporting being in the highest level of life satisfaction. It is a negative mental health effect similar to an individual losing a life partner. Being in a high-income distribution and living in a safe neighborhood are very significant aspects of high life satisfaction. Latin Americans value safety as a critical component of well-being, happiness, mental health, and life satisfaction. The increase in life satisfaction from living in very safe areas is significant and an important component of well-being above overall income in Latin America (Ortega Londoño et al., 2019).

BARRIERS TO MENTAL HEALTH CARE AND WELL-BEING IN LATIN AMERICA

One of the biggest issues for addressing mental illness and associated addiction in Latin America is stigma. Stigma refers to a characteristic that is deeply demeaning and reduces a whole person to a contaminated, devalued one. Stigma exists when aspects such as labeling, stereotyping, separating, status loss, and discrimination occur together. Stigma is a global concern but is very prevalent in Latin America for impacting treatment (Sapag et al., 2018). An effective way to tackle and address this concern is through the integration of mental health services into primary health care (PHC). At present, there has been progress in awareness and education about the occurrence of stigma. However, there is an inadequate understanding of how to prevent stigma and increase recovery-oriented practices within PHC systems. Sapag et al. (2018) reviewed 217 research articles to investigate stigma. They identified an urgent need to create interventions that understand and reduce stigma for mental health in PHC settings in Latin America (Sapag et al., 2018).

Working with PHC providers and users is an excellent intervention strategy to address this need. A recent investigation in Brazil found that 41.4% of individuals using PHC centers also suffered from some mental illness. The main obstacle to individuals receiving and accessing effective mental health care was stigma. The stigma underlying alcohol, drug use, and mental illness by society and providers were identified as a barrier to getting help. The concern over being judged by providers or others and a feeling of low self-worth as a result of getting help was identified as significant concern. Stigma training for health professionals, the creation of protocols to identify and address existing or potential stigma, and the promotion of stigma-free and recovery-focused circumstances for care were identified as possible solutions (Sapag et al., 2018).

INNOVATIVE APPROACHES FOR MENTAL HEALTH TREATMENT IN LATIN AMERICA

There is a major gap between mental health needs and access to treatment, as well as inadequate treatment of mental health conditions in Latin America. This is especially true within socioeconomically disadvantaged groups. In 2018, the average treatment gap between those suffering from mental illness and those receiving treatment for moderate to severe mental health disorders is 53.2% in North America, 74.7% in Latin America, 78.7% in Mesoamerica, and 73.1% in South America. Over 80% of children with mental illness in Latin America do not receive treatment. Mental illness is highly prevalent among children and adolescents with 16.2% in Puerto Rico, 38.3% in Chile, and 39.4% in Mexico suffering from mental health concerns. Progress to reduce the mental health treatment gap in Latin America has been slow (Kohn et al., 2018). According to the World Health Organization, mental and neurological disorders make up approximately 25% of the disease burden in Latin America and the Caribbean. A major barrier to accessing enough services is the small number of mental health professionals in the region. These are defined as psychologists, nurses, social workers, and occupational therapists. The insufficient number of mental health professionals presents a major challenge to accessibility to services (Jiménez-Molina et al., 2019).

However, internet access and smartphone use in the area has increased significantly. This major and rapid increase in internet and smartphone use can definitely help to address this gap in a variety of ways. It can be an effective platform to provide more widely distributed, low-cost mental health care in multiple situations. Jiménez-Molina et al. (2019) reviewed 22 internet-based studies in Latin America for the prevention, treatment, education, and self-care management of mental health disorders. Most of these 22 studies were conducted in Brazil, Mexico, and Chile. The researchers' analysis found that internet-based interventions for the prevention and management of mental illness are rapidly growing (Jiménez-Molina et al., 2019).

However, little research exists on the effectiveness and cost of internet-based interventions. Therefore, it is difficult to conclude whether they are effective for mental health treatment. They may be positively impactful for stigma, awareness, education, and low-level self-care support. Another important concern is the consideration of telehealth and online platforms for treatment. Studies conducted on telehealth treatment for depression in Brazil, Mexico, Colombia, and Chile seemed to achieve similar positive outcomes in symptom reduction as traditional face-to-face in-person treatment. Internet-based self-help programs were initially useful, but adherence and completion rates were low (Jiménez-Molina et al., 2019).

The evidence shows that telehealth therapy and psychiatry interventions may be an effective way to increase outpatient mental health treatment and reduce depression in a low-cost, easy-to-implement way. However, independent unguided self-help programs are less effective than asynchronous online interaction. Some glitches and issues with this included reliability and access to the internet in different regions and countries. Psychoeducational programs were attempted in Brazil using tele-education with weekly web conference seminars, but they faced significant obstacles related to internet connectivity and the use of new technology with health professionals, specifically, physicians. However, a study conducted in Brazil and Peru using mobile phones found increases in daily life activities, motivation, education on self-care, and reduction in depression symptoms as a result of mobile phone programs. Smartphones may be a positive and effective alternative for accessing more reliable and consistent internet for teletherapy support (Jiménez-Molina et al., 2019).

Internet-based interventions for mental health promotion have demonstrated benefits in high-income regions. However, these studies show they are also very effective for lower-income regions of the world and in Latin America. Internet and digital technologies improve access and create greater flexibility for mental health treatment. There is a need for further studies to assess long-term results. Specifically, school environments may be significant spaces for mental health promotion, prevention, and early detection of mental health problems. They can also be opportunities for teachers to receive greater training on mental health. The review of the literature shows that internet-based interventions are at an early stage in Latin American development. Further efforts and research are warranted in this area as a potential path for increasing mental health and well-being (Jiménez-Molina et al., 2019).

Excitingly, an increasing number of telehealth centers are being created to address this gap. Some of these programs exist in Brazil, Costa Rica, Chile, and Peru, for example. Tele-mental health is a way to reach people who would otherwise not access mental healthcare due to physical limitations or stigma. Most mental health facilities are in major cities and so tele-mental health provides increased access to care for rural residents. Another concern with receiving treatment is worry over confidentiality and reputation. In small, rural communities it is highly likely that a resident already knows the mental health provider or the provider has relationships with others that the resident knows. Therefore, this can be a barrier to even attempting treatment. Having providers based remotely outside communities through telehealth can provide a sense of safety and security to be open and seek treatment (Phillip, 2017).

However, some significant barriers in implementing telehealth services exist. One of the greatest barriers is cost, which includes the cost of a telephone, internet service, electricity, and physical structure to engage in the sessions. Another barrier is the inadequate number of mental health professionals to provide these services. A greater number would need to be recruited, which can be challenging in countries with limited higher education and training facilities in place. Another component would be training patients on receiving care using telehealth services. Lastly, intercountry coordination efforts would need to be made for licensing among mental health professionals providing treatment (Phillip, 2017). However, in spite of these barriers, tele-mental health is a potential major solution for treatment and can be accessed by much larger numbers of people in Latin America, thereby addressing a greatly needed public health concern (Phillip, 2017).

MENTAL HEALTH OF UNDERREPRESENTED GROUPS IN LATIN AMERICA

LGBTQ Groups and Mental Health in Latin America

According to Henry et al. (2021), lesbian, gay, bisexual, and transgender adults in Latin America suffer from a significantly higher level of depression and suicidal ideation than other groups. Their study found that 51.5% of the 99 participants experienced lifetime suicidal ideation. This was also associated with experiences of harassment, rejection, and discrimination. This discrimination came from family members, friends, and neighbors. It was often experienced along with violence, sexual harassment, not being hired, mistreatment by police, and threats and insults. Depression was associated with suicidal ideation in the sample. Higher levels of social support helped to function as a protective buffer for mental health concerns and, specifically, as a protective mechanism for suicidal ideation and suicide attempt (Henry et al., 2021).

Criminal Offenders and Mental Health in Latin America

A significant number of criminal offenders in Latin America struggle with mental illness and psychiatric conditions. There is a high level of need for mental health care, but the vast majority do not receive treatment. The limited research in Latin America regarding prison circumstances suggests that prison conditions are poor to extremely harsh, overcrowded, and life-threatening. The majority of these prisons do not meet international prison standards. However, in general, information on the existence of mental illness in Latin American countries is limited or unavailable. Standardized mental health services, assessments, and screening tools are lacking. Given the unusually high rates of victimization and crime in Latin America and its steady increase in the last two decades, the connection between mental illness, crime, and the prison systems should not be overlooked. More preventative, generalized mental health interventions should be made to decrease the overall health burden of mental illness. Decreasing the burden of mental illness will be assisting not only victims of crime but also offenders with mental illness to not repeat criminal behaviors and activities (Almanzar et al., 2015).

RURAL LOW-INCOME GROUPS AND MENTAL HEALTH IN LATIN AMERICA

Another underrepresented group that is worth looking at for mental health and happiness in Latin America is low-income rural groups and comparing them to urban groups. Nepomuceno et al. (2016) conducted a study in Brazil, which is one of the most economically unequal countries in the world with 16.2 million people living in extreme poverty. Nepomuceno et al. (2016) used surveys to collect sociodemographic data and ask questions from the Personal Wellbeing Index and Self Report Questionnaire (SRQ-20). The study revealed major differences between rural and urban communities regarding well-being and common mental health disorders. The researchers found a higher average well-being score in rural communities and higher levels of common mental disorders in urban environments. The prevalence of common mental disorders was found to be higher among women and strongly related to social, psychosocial, and economic circumstances (Nepomuceno et al., 2016).

The best overall average rates of mental health and well-being were found among residents in rural areas. Individuals living in big cities reported greater psychological distress. Some proposed reasons for this were increased levels of stress, coping with everyday adverse situations, weaker levels of social support, less healthy lifestyles, and challenges accessing essential goods. Psychological and social situations were more significant in understanding well-being than financial income alone in spite of extreme poverty levels. Overall, although rural areas had a higher level of poverty, well-being, and mental health were still better in rural than urban areas. The research demonstrated the significance and importance of psychosocial protective factors (Nepomuceno et al., 2016).

INDIGENOUS GROUPS AND MENTAL HEALTH IN LATIN AMERICA

Another minority group of considerable mental health and well-being concern in Latin America is the indigenous native populations. Azuero et al. (2017) reviewed 1,862 articles regarding indigenous populations and mental health in Brazil, Colombia, Chile, and Peru and found that suicide was cited as a very significant concern. High rates of suicide were believed to be a result of lifestyle changes, industrialization, environmental degradation, and alcohol. Many described these entities as a kind of cultural loss. A majority of deaths occurred through hanging or poison. High rates of alcoholism and panic attacks were other common issues among Latin American indigenous peoples. Contributing factors associated with indigenous population suicides, mental illness, and addiction included loss of original territories, climate change, modern lifestyles with high alcohol consumption, and cultural and religious subjugation. There was also a lack of mental health services and community support to address these concerns (Azuero et al., 2017).

SUMMARY

The Latin American region is a unique and unparalleled mental health and happiness phenomenon. Nowhere else in the world can one observe such a stark contrast between violence, poverty, and high levels of mental illness and, conversely, such consistently high levels of happiness that place the region in the world's top-tier happiness rankings. The region has a strong foundation in prioritizing family, psychosocial support, and happiness as important, critical values despite other life events occurring. One area that could be improved upon is strengthening community mental health services and support to address the stressors and impacts of poverty, violence, and mental illness in a more accessible way. According to Sapag, Rush & Ferris (2016), an evaluation of Latin American mental healthcare needs was conducted by providing evidence for the validity of creating a collaborative mental healthcare system (Sapag et al., 2018). Their work assessed public health networks in Mexico, Nicaragua, and Chile and involved local stakeholders. The results from their study point to the importance of creating a comprehensive framework for collaborative mental health care in Latin America. This will best support ever-changing community needs and concerns that should be addressed. It will help with identifying and evaluating ongoing mental health needs as well as changes in trends and concerns (Sapag et al., 2018). In summary, flexible, adaptable approaches need to be conducted to address the myriad of factors impacting Latin American happiness. Providing accessible, widespread community mental health services is a good way to begin to effectively tackle these concerns.

LIST OF KEY TAKEAWAYS

- Latin America has a unique happiness paradox with very high levels of mental illness, poverty, and violence, and strangely high levels of corresponding happiness and well-being.
- Psychosocial support, family, close relationships, and a priority on happiness are key protective buffers.
- Suicide and alcoholism are very significant concerns among indigenous populations in Latin America.
- Minority groups and direct survivors of violence suffer much higher levels of mental illness compared to other groups in Latin America.
- There is a major gap in mental health and violence prevention services in Latin America. Flexible, widespread community-based interventions and telehealth services are important for addressing this gap.

REVIEW QUESTIONS

- In 3 to 4 sentences, summarize a potentially effective approach to increase mental health care and happiness levels in Latin America.
- Compare and contrast the general state of mental health between 2 minority groups in the Latin American region.
- What is the Latin American happiness paradox as demonstrated in this chapter?
- What surprised you about this chapter, or what is one thing you learned that you didn't expect?

REFERENCES

Almanzar, S., Katz, C. L., & Harry, B. (2015). Treatment of mentally ill offenders in nine developing Latin American countries. *Journal of the American Academy of Psychiatry and the Law*, 43(3), 340–349. https://jaapl.org/content/43/3/340

Azuero, A. J., Arreaza-Kaufman, D., Coriat, J., Tassinari, S., Faria, A., Castañeda-Cardona, C., & Rosselli, D. (2017). Suicide in the indigenous population of Latin America: A systematic review. *Revista Colombiana de Psiquiatria*, 46(4), 237–242. https://doi.org/10.1016/j.rcp.2016.12.002

Graham, C., & Nikolova, M. (2018). Happiness and international migration in Latin America. In J. F. Helliwell, R. Layard, & J. Sachs (Eds.), *World happiness report 2018* (pp. 88–114). Sustainable Development Solutions Network. https://worldhappiness.report/ed/2018/

Helliwell, J., Layard, R., & Sachs, J. (Eds.) (2019). *World happiness report 2019*. Sustainable Development Solutions Network. https://worldhappiness.report/ed/2019/

Henry, R. S., Hoetger, C., Rabinovitch, A. E., Aguayo Arelis, A., Rabago Barajas, B. V., & Perrin, P. B. (2021). Discrimination, mental health, and suicidal ideation among sexual minority adults in Latin America: Considering the roles of social support and religiosity. *Trauma Care*, 1(3), 143–161. https://doi.org/10.3390/traumacare1030013

Jiménez-Molina, Á., Franco, P., Martínez, V., Martínez, P., Rojas, G., & Araya, R. (2019). Internet-based interventions for the prevention and treatment of mental disorders in Latin America: A scoping review. *Frontiers in Psychiatry*, 10(664). https://doi.org/10.3389/fpsyt.2019.00664

Kohn, R., Ali, A. A., Puac-Polanco, V., Figueroa, C., López-Soto, V., Morgan, K., Saldivia, S., & Vicente, B. (2018). Mental health in the Americas: An overview of the treatment gap. *Revista Panamericana de Salud Pública*, 42, e165. https://doi.org/10.26633/RPSP.2018.165

Minoletti, A., Galea, S., & Susser, E. (2012). Community mental health services in Latin America for people with severe mental disorders. *Public Health Reviews*, 34(2), 1–23. https://doi.org/10.1007/BF03391681

Nepomuceno, B. B., Cardoso, A. A. V., Ximenes, V. M., Barros, J. P. P., & Leite, J. F. (2016). Mental health, well–being, and poverty: A study in urban and rural communities in Northeastern Brazil. *Journal of Prevention & Intervention in the Community*, 44(1), 63–75. https://doi.org/10.1080/10852352.2016.1102590

Ortega Londoño, C., Gómez Mesa, D., Cardona-Sosa, L., & Gómez Toro, C. (2019). Happiness and victimization in Latin America. *Journal of Happiness Studies*, 20(3), 935–954. https://doi.org/10.1007/s10902-018-9981-3

Phillip, T. M. (2017). Telemental health in Latin America and the Caribbean. In H. Jefee-Bahloul, A. Barkil-Oteo, & E. G. Augusterfer (Eds.), *Telemental health in resource-limited global settings (pp. 181–192). Oxford University Press.*

Rojas, M. (2018). Happiness in Latin America has social foundations. In J. F. Helliwell, R. Layard, & J. Sachs (Eds.), *World happiness report 2018 (pp. 89–114).* Sustainable Development Solutions Network. https://worldhappiness.report/ed/2018/

Sapag, J. C., Sena, B. F., Bustamante, I. V., Bobbili, S. J., Velasco, P. R., Mascayano, F., Alvarado, R., & Khenti, A. (2018). Stigma towards mental illness and substance use issues in primary health care: Challenges and opportunities for Latin America. *Global Public Health*, 13(10), 1468–1480. https://doi.org/10.1080/17441692.2017.1356347

CHAPTER 4

OVERVIEW OF VARIATION IN MENTAL ILLNESS AND TREATMENT IN EUROPE

"Happiness is a new idea in Europe."
—Louis Antoine de Saint-Just

INTRODUCTION

This chapter covers the topic of mental illness, happiness, and well-being in Europe. Europe is home to the highest-ranking countries for happiness in the world, which is known as Nordic exceptionalism. However, Europe is also home to some of the highest rates of depression in many countries. There is a mix of government-sponsored mental health treatment programs in the United Kingdom, for example, as well as major treatment gaps in other areas. There is a region-wide acknowledgment of the need to provide greater mental health care through the European Mental Health Action Plan. Also, the importance of expanding government and private sector efforts with tele-psychotherapy, treating late-life depression, addressing the mental health treatment gap, and improving mental health literacy has been recognized. In addition, cultural barriers in many European countries create a stigma around accessing mental health treatment. Addressing these stigmas and overall poor mental health literacy are important steps for positive change and well-being for the whole of the region.

KEY TERMS AND DEFINITIONS

Below are common definitions and key terms that will be addressed and used throughout this book and chapter.

"Nordic Exceptionalism"

- The top five ranking countries for happiness, according to the 2020 *World Happiness Report,* are Denmark, Norway, Switzerland, Netherlands, and Sweden.
- Europe is a unique region for its great variation in well-being. It is home to the world's highest-ranking countries for happiness and well-being, which has been termed "Nordic exceptionalism," with unusually high and consistent levels of well-being (Martela, Greve, Rothstein & Saari, 2020).

European Mental Health Action Plan

- Mental health problems are among the top public health issues in the World Health Organization European Region. It is estimated that at least one-third of the European population suffers from mental illness, the most common disorders being depression and anxiety.
- The European mental health action plan was created in response to the high rates of general mental illness. It focuses on seven interconnected goals and relevant action plans to address the four priority areas of the European policy framework for health and well-being.
- Mental illness represents the greatest cause of disability and early retirement and is a significant burden to economies in Europe. This action plan represents policy action to address this significant need (World Health Organization, 2015).

Late Life Depression

- Late-life depression is a growing concern in Europe. The rising elderly population of Europe has made the mental health of older adults a larger public health issue.
- At least one-third of adults aged 65 years and older have experienced mental illness in the last year in Europe. The highest rates of late-life depression were in Southern Europe at 35%, Central and Eastern Europe at 32%, Western Europe at 26%, and Scandinavia at 17% (Horackova et al., 2019).

Overview and Background on Mental Illness, Happiness, and Treatment in Europe

As you read the section below, please consider the paradox and unique circumstances in Europe and how mental health and happiness vary in terms of significance throughout the region.

- Europe is home to the top five highest-ranking countries for happiness, mental health, and well-being in the world.
- The top five ranking countries for happiness, according to the *World Happiness Report*, are Denmark, Norway, Switzerland, Netherlands, and Sweden.
- Factors and measurements considered in well-being for Europe include mental health, physical health, income, unemployment, age, marital status, and sex.
- The ability to provide social support and have easy reporting and accessible mental health services is critical for addressing mental illness in Europe.
- Case studies such as the situation in Great Britain demonstrate the importance of easily accessible, low-cost mental health services.
- There is no downside to increasing and expanding access to mental health treatment.

It reduces the level of disability, addiction, obesity, crime, relationship deterioration, unemployment, violence, and more in society. It will eventually add up to increased wealth and development for nearly any country.

EUROPEAN MENTAL HEALTH AND TREATMENT

Europe is a unique region for its great variation in well-being. It is home to the world's highest-ranking countries for happiness and well-being, which has been termed "Nordic exceptionalism" with unusually high and consistent levels of well-being. However, Europe is also home to the top-ranking countries for depression and suicide rankings, high rates of elderly adult depression, and a huge treatment gap in mental health services (Helliwell & Wang, 2013; Helliwell et al., 2013; Layard et al., 2013).

In 2013, the top five countries for happiness, mental health, and overall well-being were Denmark, Norway, Switzerland, Netherlands, and Sweden. The bottom five were Rwanda, Burundi, Central African Republic, Benin, and Togo. The difference between the top five and bottom five is quite significant. Also, the top 10 ranking countries for mental health, well-being, and happiness in 2013 had populations below 50 million people (Helliwell & Wang, 2013; Helliwell et al., 2013; Layard et al., 2013). From 2013 until the present, the five Nordic countries of Finland, Denmark, Norway, Sweden, and Iceland, have been in the top 10 rankings for happiness and in the top three during 2017, 2018, and 2019. These Nordic states demonstrate exceptionalism in well-being that is not otherwise seen globally. It is not fully understood what accounts for this significant discrepancy between the Nordic countries and the rest of the world. However, some relevant factors that have been identified include high quality and improvement in government, autonomy, and freedom of choice, trust in others, and positive social cohesion, which are all positively associated with higher levels of well-being. The Netherlands and Switzerland, along with the Nordic countries, rank high in social support, freedom of choice, lack of government corruption, and life satisfaction (Martela et al., 2020).

In a 2013 assessment of Britain, Germany, and Australia, the factor of mental health had the greatest weight and consideration for life satisfaction and well-being. The factors that were considered in this assessment included mental health, physical health, income, unemployment, age, marital status, and sex. In these three countries, age, marital status, income, and being female decreased levels of unhappiness, and mental health problems, physical health problems, and unemployment increased unhappiness. By assessing the factors that comprise misery, which is defined as being at the bottom quarter of the population in life satisfaction, we can better understand the critical role of mental health in a population's development and progress. Mental health is the most significant variable, but due to stigma by general European populations, politicians do not adequately address the need for better mental health treatment and intervention (Helliwell & Wang, 2013; Helliwell et al., 2013; Layard et al., 2013).

WORLD HEALTH ORGANIZATION AND THE SIGNIFICANCE OF MENTAL HEALTH IN EUROPE

Mental health problems are among the top public health issues in the World Health Organization European Region. It is estimated that at least one-third of the European population suffers from mental illness, the most common disorders being depression and anxiety. Women suffer from depression twice as much as men, and 1% to 2% of the European population suffers from some form of psychosis. In addition to this, 5.6% of men and 1.3% of women are estimated to have a substance abuse disorder. However, due to poor mental health literacy and stigma, it is possible these numbers are in reality higher. Also, these numbers reflect the rates before the COVID-19 pandemic occurred (World Health Organization, 2015).

In general, the greatest amount of mental illness is found among the most vulnerable populations. Throughout the European region, neuropsychiatric disorders are the second largest cause of disease, comprising 19% of all diseases. However, there is variation, with mental illness ranking as the greatest disease burden in high-income Western European countries and fourth or fifth in low-income European countries due to high rates of perinatal and cardiovascular disease. Overall, mental disorders are the most significant chronic condition impacting Europe, making up 40% of the chronic disease burden. The number one chronic condition in Europe is depression, making up close to 14% of the total disease burden in 2015. Alcohol-related disorders comprise the second greatest disease burden. Mental disease disability accounts for some of the greatest proportion of social welfare benefits. The high rate of depression is related to suicide rates with the nine countries with the highest suicide rates in the world being in the European region. Furthermore, men are 5 times more likely to commit suicide than women in Europe, and this is related to depression, alcohol abuse, unemployment, debt, and social inequality (World Health Organization, 2015).

In response to this, there has been a commitment to deinstitutionalize mental health care and develop much greater community-based mental health treatment in Europe. The evidence shows that large mental hospitals for patients often result in neglect and institutionalization. Effective treatments for numerous mental health conditions exist that would improve well-being, and productivity, and prevent suicide. However, a great majority of individuals in Europe with mental illness never receive treatment due to inadequate accessibility, the treatment gap, and long wait times to receive treatment. The major mental health concerns in Europe include depression, anxiety, and schizophrenia. Aside from the treatment gap and poor access to mental health services, another major barrier in Europe is the problem of stigma and discrimination. If individuals engage in treatment, they often do not sufficiently maintain it due to cultural stigma and discrimination. Another barrier is negative treatment and care experiences and clients not believing treatment will help. Therefore, better training and reforms for quality mental health care may be needed. Poor mental health literacy and stigma are major barriers to care and result in individuals experiencing lower life expectancy (World Health Organization, 2015).

To address this need, a European mental health action plan was created. This action plan focuses on seven interconnected goals and relevant action plans to address the four priority areas of the European policy framework for health and well-being. As measured by prevalence, disease burden, and disability, mental illness represents the greatest cause of disability in Europe. It is also the greatest cause of early retirement and a significant burden to economies in many European countries. Thus, a policy action response is needed to address this significant concern (World Health Organization, 2015). Some of the significant goals of the European mental health action plan include:

1) All individuals have equal opportunity to achieve mental well-being, especially the most vulnerable populations;
2) Individuals with mental illness are provided full rights and consideration;
3) Mental health services are accessible, affordable, and of good quality for those in need;
4) Respectful, safe, and effective treatment is provided for all individuals in need of mental health services;
5) Good physical and mental health care is provided by health systems adequate to address the whole population;
6) Mental health systems work in conjunction and coordinated effort with other services to support a high level of care; and
7) Mental health care is informed by good knowledge and information (World Health Organization, 2015)

THE PREVALENCE OF LATE-LIFE DEPRESSION IN EUROPE

One of the most pressing mental health issues in Europe is the growing concern about late-life depression. Horackova et al. (2019) investigated the prevalence of late-life depression and the gap in mental health services in four European regions, including Western Europe, Scandinavia, Southern Europe, and Central Europe and Eastern Europe. Their research explored sociodemographic, social- and health-related factors associated with late-life depression. The population-based sample was comprised of 28,796 individuals living in Europe. Among the sample, 29% of individuals identified as suffering from late-life depression. The highest rates of late-life depression occurred in Southern Europe at 35%, Central and Eastern Europe at 32%, Western Europe at 26%, and Scandinavia at 17%. The variables with the greatest association for depression were the total number of chronic diseases, pain, daily living mobility, strength, and cognitive limitations. Among the collective sample from the four regions, there was a 79% gap in mental health service use. This means that there is a high rate of late-life depression throughout all of Europe and an overwhelmingly high gap in treatment (Horackova et al., 2019).

The growing elderly population of Europe has made the mental health of older adults a larger public health issue. At least one-third of adults aged 65 years and older have experienced mental illness in the last year in Europe. Depression is a leading cause of disability in the world and is also significant for its impact on physical and cognitive decline, reduced quality of life, and increased mortality. The work of Horackova and colleagues (2019) highlights the importance of interventions that address late-life depression and depression screenings for older adults with chronic somatic comorbidities and limited mental and physical functioning. In addition to this, interventions that decrease the stigmatization of mental illness for older adults in Europe are also worthwhile to address the mental healthcare gap in treatment (Horackova et al., 2019).

Late-life depression is the result of multiple factors; however, depression in early life predisposes an individual to a higher likelihood of depression as an adult. Socioeconomic factors and genetics seem to be important influences for younger groups in Europe; for older adults, additional factors such as frequency of social meetings, marital status, and contact with children and grandchildren are significant. Late-life depression and depression in general in Europe have a strong association with chronic illness, diseases such as cancer and cardiovascular disease, and cognitive impairment. Smoking, alcohol abuse, and physical inactivity also exacerbate and can be associated with these conditions. Depression in older adults may be more difficult to treat throughout all four regions in Europe than in younger adults. In Europe, multilayered approaches that apply psychosocial, medical, and pharmacological treatment are helpful. This is because there is a major gap in identifying individuals in need of mental health treatment as a whole throughout Europe and then connecting those who are identified with treatment. Primary medical care is a critical point of contact with individuals and particularly the elderly in Europe to identify depression, connect to treatment, and thereby improve quality of life and prevent elderly suicide (Horackova et al., 2019).

In Europe, another important factor is that older adults are less likely than younger adults to recognize the signs of depression and/or believe they have a need for mental health treatment. In addition, it is also challenging because the symptoms of late-life depression in the elderly may differ from what is seen in younger populations, particularly for those with pre-existing, comorbid conditions. No significant study in Europe has taken factors such as elderly fatigue, cognitive impairment, apathy, and other signs of mental illness into account for screening. The 79% gap in mental health services identified in this study is much higher than the global norm for treatment gaps. In addition to this, it is estimated that approximately 56% of the global population of individuals 15 years or older who have depression lack access to mental health care (Horackova et al., 2019).

THE TREATMENT GAP IN EUROPE

One of the greatest issues for well-being in Europe is the treatment gap. This is the discrepancy between the identified need for quality mental healthcare services and the actual provided services. It is estimated that there is approximately a 79% gap between those in Europe in need of mental health care services and those receiving services. Put another way, only about 20% of those needing mental health services actually receive some sort of assistance in Europe. Treatment for mental illness has important implications for life expectancy, quality of life, and the burden of disability. For example, admittance to the hospital for mental health reasons improves life expectancy by an estimated 15 to 20 years. This treatment gap has severe consequences for society. Untreated mental illness creates major costs to society that come not only in monetary form but also through strained use of the healthcare system, lost productivity, education underachievement, increased levels of violence, addiction, crime, less effective use of resources, breakdown of social and family relationships, worsening physical health and obesity, and lower overall development of human and societal potential (Helliwell & Wang, 2013; Helliwell et al., 2013; Layard et al., 2013).

Despite its demonstrated significance for health, economic, and societal outcomes, no country in the world spends more than 15% of its health budget on mental healthcare. The outliers that spend closest to 15% include England and Wales, and they have witnessed significant improvements in recent years and cost due to disability as a result of increased access and use of mental health services and government financing. There are low-cost and effective mental health treatments available that can be made much more widely available. It is illogical to not incorporate mental healthcare further into a country's budget when we see so many significant positive impacts on numerous quantifiers for development and wealth (Helliwell & Wang, 2013; Helliwell et al., 2013; Layard et al., 2013).

COVID, MENTAL HEALTH, AND HAPPINESS IN EUROPE

Another factor impacting European mental health and happiness is the influence COVID has had on overall well-being, happiness, and mental health statistics. The coronavirus pandemic significantly exacerbated symptoms of anxiety, depression, and stress as a whole in Europe. In addition, the European regions saw a significant increase in domestic violence, divorce, and suicide rates during the pandemic. This was not only a physical health crisis but also a mental health crisis in Europe, the effects of which are still being experienced. COVID helped highlight underlying mental health conditions that had been untreated and/or worsened pre-existing mental illnesses for families and individuals (Veer et al., 2020). A cross-sectional survey taken in the United Kingdom during the COVID pandemic outbreak identified significant declines in mental health, decreased happiness levels, and increases in anxiety. Cohort studies across the world also found increased levels of psychological distress and clinically significant mental illness that were reported during the first few weeks of the lockdown. However, in spite of these heightened levels of mental illness during the pandemic, some mental health estimates show that mental illness had already been worsening prior to COVID-19. Therefore, there was already a poor and declining foundation for good mental health in the United Kingdom, as well as other parts of Europe, before the pandemic even occurred (Banks et al., 2021).

This declining foundation is partly evidenced by heightened numbers of crisis and counseling calls in Europe. Research in Germany from 2020–2021, found that the number of telephone calls to Germany's largest online and telephone counseling helpline service increased by 20% in the first week of the COVID lockdown. Increased levels of loneliness, anxiety, and suicidal ideation were associated with this increased frequency in telephone calls. German states that imposed stricter lockdown measures saw a greater decline in mental health. Switzerland, in contrast, had more relaxed lockdown measures and did not see an increase in mental health crisis calls during the pandemic (Banks et al., 2021).

Potential mental health resilience factors in relation to the coronavirus epidemic were investigated by Veer and colleagues (2020) in a study of 5,000 European adults. In this study, resilience was classified as good mental health regardless of stressor exposure. The research identified the greatest negative stressors as corona-related media coverage, the inability to participate in leisure activities, loss of social contact, and feeling restricted to leave home. Some of the most significant mental health stressors were not being able to attend the funeral of a loved one, not being able to go to the hospital when a loved one was ill, and fear about loved ones becoming severely ill from COVID. Individuals with past or present mental health conditions were at greater risk of worse mental illness than individuals with no history of mental illness. However, better mental health was reported by individuals with a positive appraisal of their own circumstance and their society and reflected in higher levels of optimism. Another important factor identified for good mental health was positive stress response recovery. Mental health can be improved by focusing on and creating positive, constructive attitudes and perspectives toward circumstances (Veer et al., 2020).

CASE STUDY OF ITALY WITH COVID

Italy is an important case study for European mental health and well-being since the coronavirus epidemic. It was the first country highly impacted by the coronavirus. On March 11, 2020, the Italian government implemented an extended lockdown in response to the COVID crisis. The mental health consequences were particularly severe from COVID and government restrictions. Disabled individuals, psychiatric patients, caregivers, the elderly with chronic health concerns, and individuals in a lower socioeconomic level were most negatively impacted by their mental health. In addition to a worsened mental health environment, mental health services were also not available in Italy due to the lockdowns (Marazziti et al., 2020).

A study of 5,683 individuals conducted during the first week of COVID quarantine in Italy found that more than 40% of participants suffered from high psychological distress. Women and adults younger than 30 years of age reported higher levels of high distress with approximately 30% of individuals demonstrating posttraumatic stress symptoms. The extended lockdown was fairly effective in reducing COVID cases during the acute stage of COVID-19. However, long-term psychosocial consequences were not adequately addressed in the emergency, post-emergency, and post-pandemic phases. The coronavirus pandemic brought to light inadequacies in the Italian public healthcare system for addressing mental illness. During the time of the COVID pandemic, the Italian public healthcare system lacked community programs and sufficient investments to address mental health concerns. In addition to this, the general population as a whole had poor mental health knowledge and understanding, which contributed to ongoing mental illness concerns (Marazziti et al., 2020).

Solutions Resulting from the Italy Case Study

The Italian mental health crisis due to COVID-19 brought to light some potential solutions that could be implemented on a large scale. Not only did the Italian healthcare system have an inadequate number of mental health providers at the start of the pandemic, it also reduced its number of country-wide medical staff. The community health services were inadequate, and the pay was inadequate even for practicing medical health providers (Marazziti et al., 2020). However, appropriate mindfulness skills have been found to reduce post-traumatic stress symptoms in the Italian population. Marazziti and colleagues (2020) reported that implementing mindfulness-based interventions and programs to address large-scale mental illness needs is an effective policy approach. This is particularly true for vulnerable populations and large-scale sustainable interventions for post-pandemic care and support. The Italian public health system had an inadequate number of mental health professionals during the pandemic, and improvements can be still made post-pandemic (Marazziti et al., 2020).

Some positive occurrences in Italy that are noteworthy for treatment and for general care in Europe include the creation of a search engine called the #psicologionline, which is promoted by the National Council of the Order of Psychologists, the Italian Psychoanalytical Society, and the Italian Society of Behavioral and Cognitive Therapy. This search engine provides support to help Italians find the closest psychologist/psychotherapist near them and schedule a free consultation by telehealth. There is a need for more services than this; however, it is a positive start to addressing long-term health needs and sets an example for other European nations (Marazziti et al., 2020).

TELE-PSYCHOTHERAPY

Another potential solution to the gap in mental health treatment in Europe is tele-psychotherapy. This has become much more apparent since the COVID-19 pandemic. The use of tele-psychotherapy and online interventions, such as psychoeducation that apply psychological theories and techniques to address mental and physical health needs, has grown dramatically. Telehealth and mental health interventions through online sources are a way to navigate challenges in receiving traditional psychological care. Telehealth is not always ideal if clients find it challenging to access a private space or find enough time for an uninterrupted session. COVID-19 created a turning point for telehealth with mental health services. Types of telehealth with mental health services include internet-based interventions, smartphone apps, wearables, and virtual reality. COVID-19 saw a surge in mental health issues coming to the forefront and a heightened demand for alternative forms of treatment. In Europe, this surge of mental health issues was recognized, and the project group on e-health of the European Federation of Psychologists Associations advocated for the adoption of e-mental health technology (Van Daele et al., 2020).

IMPROVED HEALTHCARE AND SOCIAL SUPPORT FOR THE MENTALLY ILL

Additional solutions to address the European mental health situation since the COVID pandemic are improved healthcare and social support for mentally ill adults. However, as 50% of mentally ill adults experienced their mental illness by the age of 15, an even more effective approach may be early intervention with mental health services for children, adolescents, and young adults. A British study that began in the 1970s followed a cohort of British citizens born in the 1970s and followed their development at ages 5, 10, and 16, looking at emotional, behavioral, and intellectual concerns. Maintaining the levels of economic, social, and psychological factors as constants so they did not function as confounding variables, this study clearly demonstrated that the emotional development of the child is the most important variable for their life satisfaction levels as an adult. Specifically, the most effective way to have high life satisfaction levels as an adult is to have good mental health starting as a child and throughout the life span. Mental health during the formative years for children is a critical component of their development and potentially stops mental illness that would lead to low life satisfaction and poorer outcomes as an adult (Helliwell & Wang, 2013; Helliwell et al., 2013; Layard et al., 2013).

MENTAL HEALTH PROGRESS IN EUROPE

The field of mental healthcare has progressed significantly since the 1950s when the treatments available were extremely limited and torn between kind, compassionate care and more draconian residential psych ward treatments. However, since the 1950s, significant breakthroughs were made through new medications that help with depression, anxiety, bipolar, and psychotic disorders. In the 1970s, new evidenced-based therapy interventions were created including cognitive behavior therapy (CBT). It was discovered in the 1970s that up to 16 CBT sessions created similar recovery rates as medication did, with lower relapse than medication. With anxiety disorders, treatment with CBT and medication provides recovery rates of more than 50%. Therapy and drug interventions are inexpensive compared with treatment and intervention for a majority of individuals living with physical illness. When the larger cost of disability is considered, increasing wider access to psychological therapy reduces the gross cost to the public sector to zero. The research shows that there is no downside to increasing and expanding access to mental health treatment. If it reduces the level of disability, addiction, obesity, crime, relationship deterioration, unemployment, violence, and more, it will eventually add up to increased wealth and development for any country. This includes high-, middle-, and low-income regions (Helliwell & Wang, 2013; Helliwell et al., 2013; Layard et al., 2013).

This data and an understanding of the importance of mental health treatment and the overall positive impact it will have not only on society but on economics led the British government to conduct a novel program in 2008 until present to increase access to therapy. This program is called Improving Access to Psychological Therapies (IAPT) and was an innovative and impressive initiative that the government took, based on sound data and evidence. As of 2013, the program served more than half a million people a year and continues to expand. The outcomes and rates of recovery are seen to be similar to that of clinical trials. These recovery rates are also reflected in these individuals being able to consistently maintain employment and not go on government disability. The success of Britain's expanded government-backed therapy initiative helped Chile to consider implementing a similar program (Helliwell & Wang, 2013; Helliwell et al., 2013; Layard et al., 2013).

CHILD MENTAL ILLNESS

Aside from expanded access and lower cost of mental health services, another important consideration to reduce the burden of mental illness is addressing child mental illness. At least 50% of child mental illness is expressed by age 15. Child mental illness can be understood as the internalizing disorders that express themselves through anxiety and depression and externalizing disorders with behavior issues such as conduct disorder and attention-deficit hyperactivity disorder (ADHD). The evidence from clinical trials and larger government initiatives demonstrates that anxiety has 50% to 60% recovery rates with psychological therapy. Depression is effectively treated with CBT, interpersonal therapy, and medication with significant success rates. Conduct disorder, when mild to moderate in severity and with parent training, is treatable, and ADHD has a 70% recovery rate with the psychostimulant medication Methylphenidate. The data clearly demonstrate that early treatment with children is very effective as well as economically intelligent (Helliwell & Wang, 2013; Helliwell et al., 2013; Layard et al., 2013).

PREVENTION

Another component is not only early treatment but also prevention. By preventing the main risk factors that lead to mental illness, we can reduce the overall burden to society and the need to significantly expand treatment. The individual attributes that put a person at risk for mental illness include low self-esteem, emotional immaturity, trouble with communication, medical illness, and substance abuse. Social circumstances that put one at risk for mental illness include loneliness, bereavement, neglect, family conflict, exposure to violence/abuse, low income and poverty, difficulties or failure at school, and work stress or unemployment. Environmental factors that significantly impact mental health include poor access to basic services, injustice and discrimination, and exposure to war or disaster. Any or all combinations of these can lead to the development of mental illness in an individual (Helliwell & Wang, 2013; Helliwell et al., 2013; Layard, et al., 2013).

Early intervention programs and mental health initiatives serve as protective or preventive factor in developing mental illness. Some interventions can be conducted by community members through psychoeducational interventions for pregnant mothers and parents with young children. Interventions that are implemented in home, work, community, and school-based environments are effective for addressing needs. The stigma and misunderstanding about mental health may preclude individuals from accessing or trying to access mental health services aside from limitations in service provision and cost. This psychosocial support through education and public health measures may be an effective method to address multiple variables that put an individual at risk for developing a mental illness or learning how to manage early symptoms (Helliwell & Wang, 2013; Helliwell et al., 2013; Layard et al., 2013).

At its core, the greatest issue with mental health and treatment in Europe is the view, literacy, and attitude toward mental health. The attitude and stigma on mental health treatment and access is a major barrier that prevents politicians and policymakers from implementing new mental health treatment interventions. A positive change in attitude toward mental health treatment would make a significant difference in many aspects of well-being in Europe. Treatment for mental health, as evidenced by the data, is as important as physical health. In more developed countries, the groups being most overlooked are those with anxiety and depression disorders as well as children with behavioral disorders. Left without treatment, these conditions will further develop and lead to greater levels of disability and societal issues than is necessary (Helliwell & Wang, 2013; Helliwell et al., 2013; Layard et al., 2013).

Some ways to further address these concerns are educating primary healthcare providers to be much better trained to identify and treat mental illness. More than this, a new and larger group of mental health therapists may need to be created with accessibility at the same level as other medical services and community health workers. The greatest overall barrier to effective mental health treatment is, in many ways, worldwide stigma and beliefs about mental illness. This attitude and collective denial or suppression of the issue only worsens, not helps damage to individuals and society as a whole. The World Health Assembly Comprehensive Mental Health Action Plan signifies a political commitment for countries worldwide to improve mental health and address this stigma head-on (Helliwell & Wang, 2013; Helliwell et al., 2013; Layard et al., 2013). It is worthwhile for Europe to implement and take consistent action on this commitment.

LIST OF KEY TAKEAWAYS

- The European region presents a contrast in that the Nordic countries rank among the top 10 "happiest" countries in the world while the 9 countries with the highest suicide rates are also in Europe.
- Poor mental health literacy and stigma are major barriers to effective mental health care.
- Depression is the greatest mental health concern and the greatest overall health issue in Europe.
- Telehealth, mindfulness-based interventions, and psychoeducation offer unique opportunities to address prevalent mental illness concerns in Europe.
- There is a significant mental health treatment gap for all groups, but especially for the most vulnerable in Europe.

REVIEW QUESTIONS

- In 3 to 4 sentences, summarize a potentially effective approach to improve mental health care and happiness levels in Europe.
- Compare and contrast the general state of mental health in the elderly adult population in Europe to the general population.
- What presents as the greatest disease burden in the European region?
- What surprised you about this chapter, or what is one thing you learned that you didn't expect?

REFERENCES

Banks, J., Fancourt, D., & Xu, X. (2021). Mental health and the COVID-19 pandemic. In J. F. Helliwell, R. Layard, J. Sachs, & J-E. De Neve (Eds.), *World happiness report 2021 (pp.107–130).* Sustainable Development Solutions Network. https://happiness-report.s3.amazonaws.com/2021/WHR+21.pdf

Helliwell, J., Layard, R., & Sachs, J. (Eds.) (2013). *World happiness report 2013.* Sustainable Development Solutions Network. *https://worldhappiness.report/ed/2013/*

Helliwell, J. F., & Wang, S. (2013). World happiness: Trends, explanations and distribution. In J. Helliwell, R. Layard, & J. Sachs (Eds.), *World happiness report 2013. Sustainable Development Solutions Network. https://worldhappiness.report/ed/2013/*

Horackova, K., Kopecek, M., Machů, V., Kagstrom, A., Aarsland, D., Motlova, L. B., & Cermakova, P. (2019). Prevalence of late-life depression and gap in mental health service use across European regions. *European Psychiatry, 57,* 19–25. https://doi.org/10.1016/j.eurpsy.2018.12.002

Layard, R., Chisholm, D., Patel, V., & Saxena, S. (2013). Mental illness and unhappiness. (Discussion Paper No. 1239) Center for Economic Performance, London School of Economics and Political Science. https://cep.lse.ac.uk/pubs/download/dp1239.pdf

Marazziti, D., Pozza, A., Di Giuseppe, M., & Conversano, C. (2020). The psychosocial impact of COVID-19 pandemic in Italy: A lesson for mental health prevention in the first severely hit European country. *Psychological Trauma: Theory, Research, Practice, and Policy, 12(*5), 531–533. https://doi.org/10.1037/tra0000687

Martela, F., Greve, B., Rothstein, B., & Saari, J. (2020). The Nordic exceptionalism: What explains why the Nordic countries are constantly among the happiest in the world. In J. Helliwell, R. Layard, & J. Sachs (Eds.), *World happiness report 2020* (pp. 129–146). *Sustainable Development Solutions Network. https://worldhappiness.report/ed/2020/*

Van Daele, T., Karekla, M., Kassianos, A. P., Compare, A., Haddouk, L., Salgado, J., Ebert, D. D., Trebbi, G., Bernaerts, S., Van Assche, E., & De Witte, N. A. (2020). Recommendations for policy and practice of telepsychotherapy and e-mental health in Europe and beyond. *Journal of Psychotherapy Integration, 30(*2), 160–173. https://doi.org/10.1037/int0000218

Veer, Riepenhausen, A., Zerban, M., Wackerhagen, C., Engen, H., Puhlmann, L. M. C., Köber, G., van Leeuwen, J., Tüscher, O., Yuen, K. S. L., Walter, H., & Kalisch, R. (2020). Mental resilience to stressor prevalence and severity during the Corona lockdown in Europe. *Psychoneuroendocrinology, 119,* 104984–. https://doi.org/10.1016/j.psyneuen.2020.104984

World Health Organization. (2015). *The European mental health action plan 2013–2020.* World Health Organization. Regional Office for Europe. https://apps.who.int/iris/handle/10665/175672

CHAPTER 5

MENTAL HEALTH IN SUB-SAHARAN AFRICA

Two things define you—your attitude when you have everything,
your patience when you have nothing.

—Igbo African Elders

INTRODUCTION

This chapter provides an in-depth overview of mental health, well-being, and happiness in sub-Saharan Africa. The beginning of the chapter offers an overview of mental health and treatment in sub-Saharan Africa. It discusses challenges in conducting research in Africa, research breakthroughs, and successful initiatives. Demographic changes in the region are explored as well as current trends and predictions for rising population, mental illness, and substance abuse rates. Resiliency and protective factors, innovative solutions, and interventions are explored. Current and projected trends regarding mental health, well-being, and happiness are discussed as well as key takeaways.

KEY TERMS AND DEFINITIONS

Below are common definitions and key terms that will be addressed and used throughout this book and chapter.

Sub-Saharan African Optimism

- The cultural belief in many cultures in sub-Saharan Africa is that regardless of current circumstances, the future will inevitably improve.
- A noted pervasive and unusual level of optimism among youth in sub-Saharan Africa serves as a protective, resiliency factor in mental health and well-being.
- This optimism tends to decrease with age but serves as a positive protective mechanism despite challenging sociodemographic conditions (Helliwell et al., 2017; Møller et al., 2017).

Happiness Deficit

- The relative gap in well-being, mental health, and happiness a group or region experiences in comparison to other worldwide, measured norms
- According to the 2017 World Happiness Report, compared to other regions of the world, Africa has a "happiness deficit" that is quite large.
- The known levels of happiness are much lower in the African region than in most other regions of the world, however, there is also a paucity of mental health and well-being data available in this region (Møller et al., 2017).

Resilience

- The ability to recover quickly, manage, and withstand great challenges, stress, difficulties, emotional upheaval, and suffering.
- The sub-Saharan African continent has widespread levels of resilience through the practice of patience, acceptance, culturally-embedded coping skills, and resourcefulness (Møller & Roberts, 2021).

Overview

- The 2017 *World Happiness Report* presents an important emphasis on African happiness and demonstrates a *happiness deficit* that is specific to this region.
- There have been challenges in obtaining adequate research on happiness, mental health, and well-being in Africa as a whole. However, an increasing number of studies and initiatives are being employed to gather reliable data.
- Unique resilience and protective factors such as optimism and religiosity in many African cultures help with managing mental health and substance use concerns.
- Africa is going through a significant change in population and regional health currently that is expected to continue well into the foreseeable future.
- In recent years, Africa has leapfrogged in technology advancements with greater widespread access to mobile phones and solar-powered electricity.
- It is a region with a tumultuous and unique history, ideas, and beliefs. and perceptions of well-being and happiness may be different from other regions of the world as every African country is different, and within each country, there is an abundance of cultural diversity.

MENTAL HEALTH AND TREATMENT IN SUB-SAHARAN AFRICA

The 2017 *World Happiness Report* presents an important emphasis on African happiness. Africa is comprised of 54 countries. It is a huge landmass and home to the largest number of nation-states on one continent. Africa consists of such a large number of countries that it makes up 47 of the 166 countries in the Gallup World Poll or approximately a quarter of all countries. The *World Happiness Report* tracks the happiness of 44 out of 54 African countries and is a reliable indicator for data and insight into the current and trending situation regarding the region's well-being. Africa is a unique continent as it has the longest-known history of humankind with a huge mix of cultural, language, and ethnic variety. It has a history of centuries of slavery, colonialism, and apartheid before independence. African people have adopted some of the customs, technological advances, and lifestyles of former colonial rulers (Møller et al., 2017).

Most recently, Africa has leapfrogged with technology advancements through mobile phones and solar-powered electricity. Given its tumultuous and unique history, its ideas, and beliefs. and perceptions of well-being and happiness may be different from other regions of the world. Each country in Africa is different, and within each is cultural diversity. According to the 2017 *World Happiness Report*, compared to other regions of the world, Africa has a "happiness deficit" that is quite apparent in contrast to the rest of the world. This means that the levels of happiness are much lower here than in most other regions of the world (Møller et al., 2017).

Research Challenges

However, even though a conclusion was drawn regarding a happiness deficit in Africa, there is a paucity of data regarding mental health and well-being on the continent. The data from the 2017 *World Happiness Report* that made the happiness deficit conclusion was obtained from the Afrobarometer. The Afrobarometer collects information on subjective indicators for the average individual on the continent of Africa. There is a dearth of information on subjective indicators for the continent of Africa as a whole. Most studies focus on specific subregions such as sub-Saharan Africa, North Africa, and/or the Middle East, and not the entire continent. This shortage of data makes it challenging to understand the mental health and well-being of populations living on the continent as a whole. Also, some research that has been conducted reported higher levels of happiness than were accurate due to cultural misunderstandings (Helliwell et al., 2017; Møller, et al., 2017).

Some research on the continent of Africa found that individuals reported being "happy" despite mental illness, family concerns, unemployment, and health circumstances. This was clearly demonstrated in research in Nigeria where the happiness paradox was identified. In Nigeria, respondents were questioned about their mental health and well-being. These respondents reported being happier than they actually were. By reporting higher levels of happiness, they meant to avoid further stress and problems in their lives and counteract negative life circumstances. In essence, reporting higher than true levels of well-being was indicative of high levels of denials and coping. On the whole, false positivity was a suppression and coping mechanism for managing well-being when other resources were unavailable. Low levels of subjective well-being are not likely to be a new phenomenon in Africa. The earliest international studies on happiness found lower levels of well-being and mental health south of the Sahara than was found in most regions of the world (Helliwell et al., 2017; Møller et al., 2017).

The Gallup World Poll and Hadley Cantril

The Gallup World Poll is an important measurement tool to understand global levels of well-being. It was introduced in 2005 and is conducted in approximately 140 countries every year worldwide. It is carried out in 40 countries on the continent of Africa and surveys about 1,000 residents per country. The goal of the Gallup World Poll is to produce relevant data that apply to the whole civilian, noninstitutionalized population aged 15 years or older. Face-to-face surveys are conducted as much as possible. In regions such as Libya, where it has been dangerous to conduct face-to-face surveys, telephone surveys have been implemented to obtain data. Certain countries are too difficult to obtain consistent data such as Nigeria, Somalia, and South Sudan where insecurity makes it very dangerous to conduct interviews. Low levels of well-being were noted in studies conducted in the 1960s using the ladder of life measure from Hadley Cantril, which looked at 13 countries worldwide including two African countries. This research found low levels of mental health and well-being in the African region (Helliwell et al., 2017; Møller et al., 2017).

Another study, the Gallup-Kettering study, was also significant for finding unusually low levels of well-being in the African region. It was conducted in the 1970s and was the largest global study on mental health and well-being of its time. In this study, Africa ranked at the lowest levels of well-being worldwide aside from India. The Gallup-Kettering study also looked at the connection between mental health and the desire for change. Specifically, 90% of African respondents reported that their levels of well-being, mental health, and happiness would significantly increase if many things could change in their lives (Helliwell et al., 2017; Møller et al., 2017).

In addition to this, early research also points to the importance and association between effective, good governance and well-being. There is a strong connection between well-being, good governance, and positive mental health. Decreased satisfaction with democracy is associated with decreased levels of happiness. The research demonstrates that Africans view democracy as not only having free and fair elections but also better living conditions such as clean water, electricity, housing, and the freedom to criticize the government (Helliwell et al., 2017; Møller, et al., 2017).

Lived Poverty and Happiness

The Gallup World Poll demonstrates that lived poverty (found in the Afrobarometer Lived Poverty Index) is an important factor in mental health and well-being measurements. A case study of Zimbabwe demonstrates the relationship between poverty and insecurity with mental health and happiness. The greater the drop in poverty scores, the higher the corresponding happiness and well-being score (Helliwell et al., 2017; Møller et al., 2017).

From 2005 to 2015, the Gallup World Poll found a relationship between levels of lived poverty and happiness for data collected from Botswana, South Africa, Uganda, Tanzania, Madagascar, Ghana, Namibia, Mali, Benin, Zimbabwe, Nigeria, Zambia, Malawi, Senegal, and Kenya. In addition to lived poverty levels and good governance on the continent of Africa, an important part of happiness, well-being, and mental health is infrastructure development. The Afrobarometer identified that, on average, in only two thirds of 35 countries do people live in communities with an electric grid (65%) and/or piped water (63%). Fewer than 30% have access to sewage services in contrast to 93% of the population having access to cellular phone service. Aside from this, only about half, or 54%, live in a region with tarred or paved roads. In contrast to sub-Saharan Africa, North Africa has the best infrastructure and highest access to electricity, piped water, sewage services, paved roads, and cellular phone service. North Africa also has the highest average happiness, mental health, and well-being scores compared to the rest of the African continent (Helliwell et al., 2017; Møller et al., 2017).

The Case of South Africa

South Africa provides an enlightening picture of happiness and well-being between the poorer black South Africans in contrast to the wealthier white South Africans. Indicators for mental health, well-being, and happiness for poorer black South Africans point to the significance of infrastructure and public goods. By contrast, the indicators for mental health and happiness for wealthier white South Africans are associated with indicators identified in Western, more developed research settings (Helliwell et al., 2017; Møller et al., 2017).

The Rise of Technology and Current Trends

This section discusses the role of age gaps in leadership, issues of unemployment, climate change, and population growth in relation to mental health and wellness in the African region. Increases in technology and current events and trends play an important role in these issues of concern, and will likely be relevant for future policymakers.

Age Gap of Leadership. A lesser commonly identified mental health and happiness component is the age gap between Africa's leaders and the general population. About 70% of the general population in Africa is less than 30 years of age whereas most of Africa's leaders are 70 years or more. Many of these leaders lived during the colonial era and before television, the internet, and cellular phones. The vast majority of the population may have difficulty trusting or relating to these leaders and feel like their needs and concerns are being met. A significant and interesting development in Africa is the rapid growth of mobile-cellular phones and widespread internet use. The rates of their growth are close to that of the rest of the world, and the technologies offer a potential tool for addressing mental health and happiness in new and innovative ways (Helliwell et al., 2017; Møller et al., 2017).

Unemployment. The most recent Afrobarometer found that unemployment is a high-level concern for African countries, and improvements in education and employment could make a considerable improvement in mental health and happiness levels. The 2016 Afrobarometer reported that 38% of respondents in a survey of 36 countries\ identified unemployment as the most significant concern impacting well-being and mental health. This was followed by 32% of respondents saying that health was one of the most important problems (Helliwell et al., 2017; Møller et al., 2017).

Climate Change and Population Growth. Other significant components of happiness, mental health, and well-being in Africa are the issues of drought, extreme weather patterns, and rising population rates. This has only been further aggravated by global warming. Drought and extreme weather negatively impact infrastructure development, food production, health, economic growth, good governance, and societal stability. A greater focus on investing in Africa's youth could make a significant difference in addressing all of the above issues. Africa struggles with a population challenge in that it had been underpopulated for many centuries but now experiences a population explosion (Helliwell et al., 2017; Møller et al., 2017).

Africa's population is expected to double by 2050, and this has put severe pressure and caused significant challenges to the state to provide education, health services, infrastructure, and the capacity to address other essential needs. The population explosion combined with the impact of global warming may undermine the human development progress that Africa has experienced. This decline in development is projected to lead to worsening mental health, happiness, and well-being levels. As of 2016, 78% of African countries have not transitioned into a demographic change that includes low fertility and low mortality. The countries with the highest fertility rates globally are all in sub-Saharan Africa with more than 6 children per woman. This high fertility rate, large youth population, and foundation of other challenges may lead to significant concerns in well-being in the future for African residents (Helliwell et al., 2017; Møller et al., 2017).

Adolescent Mental Health and Happiness

Sub-Saharan Africa has the most rapidly growing adolescent population in the world. The health and socioeconomic challenges adolescents in this region face increase their risk of poor mental health. The most common issues adolescents experience includes depression, anxiety, and post-traumatic stress disorder. The stigma associated with mental illness and inadequate understanding of the connection between mental health and poverty means these issues have been given less attention by policymakers. Traditional healers may be the most accessible form of care for help-seeking adolescents (Sequeira et al., 2022).

There are considerable levels of mental illness among children and adolescents in sub-Saharan Africa. One in 7 children and adolescents have major challenges and at least 1 in 10 have a significant psychiatric condition. Socio-demographics are shown to have a major impact on the children with the greatest deprivation at the highest risk for mental illness. Eleven community-based studies in sub-Saharan Africa were meta-analyzed to better understand the psychopathology of children ages 0 to 16 years. It is increasingly recognized that mental health is a critical aspect of child development. Psychological challenges significantly impact a child's ability to reach their full potential. Psychological disorders in adults are a particularly large issue in sub-Saharan Africa. Posttraumatic stress disorder, anxiety, and depression are estimated to be at 20% to 60% among adults. There are 48 countries in sub-Saharan Africa, and they comprise the largest group of the least-developed countries worldwide (Cortina et al., 2012).

Improving child psychosocial well-being is necessary to attain children's potential and attain United Nations' millennium development goals. It is estimated that depression alone will become the single largest disease burden for all health conditions by 2030. It is estimated that 1 in 7 children and adolescents struggle with their mental health and 1 in 10 have a diagnosable psychiatric disorder. A systematic review that looked at children ages 0 to 16 years assessed data from 9,713 children in six countries and found that 14.3% of the children identified as having some type of psychopathology. Some estimates predicted close to 20% of identified populations had psychopathology; other estimates were closer to 10%. On the whole, this demonstrates the importance of increasing awareness and identification of mental health in Africa (Cortina et al., 2012). Other conditions such as post-traumatic stress disorder, anxiety, and depression are of important concern to adults with rates estimated at 20% to 60% of the adult population. The greatest proportion of the least developed countries in the world comes from 48 sub-Saharan countries. Adverse childhood experiences may interfere with fundamental child physical, emotional, and social developmental needs. These adverse childhood experiences put them at risk for psychological problems. Mental health problems are common in sub-Saharan Africa in individuals ages 0 to 16 years old. The disorders most often identified in this review include emotional problems such as depression, anxiety, conduct, disruptive, reactive behavior disorders as well as posttraumatic stress disorder (Cortina et al., 2012).

THE GROWTH OF IDENTIFIED MENTAL ILLNESS IN SUB-SAHARAN AFRICA

Sub-Saharan Africa has historically had a focus on diseases related to poverty that are connected to concerns such as malnutrition, unclean water, and infectious disease. However, worldwide there is a major shift occurring with an aging population and disease burden increasingly reflected in chronic illness and disability through mental health concerns such as depression. Yet, predictive health models suggest that during the next 40 years, sub-Saharan Africa will witness reduced mortality and a major spike in chronic disease as a result. The population of sub-Saharan Africa is expected to double in the next 40 years from .9 billion to 1.8 billion with a growing aging population than previously experienced. These estimates come from the Global Burden of Disease 2010 study data and UN population predictions. These data predict that population growth and aging will lead to an estimated 130% increase in the burden of mental health and substance use disorders by 2050 in sub-Saharan Africa. This predicted surge in mental illness and substance use disorders is projected to have significant negative impacts on health and productivity (Charlson et. al, 2014).

As a result of this, there is a need to work ahead and create the infrastructure necessary to address these concerns. An estimated increase of at least 216,000 mental health workers is required in sub-Saharan Africa by 2050. Some solutions to this heightened need include a significant investment in training primary care practitioners, improving community mental health resources, and expanding inpatient psychiatric units available in the community and urban general hospitals. The biggest projected concerns are depression, alcohol, and opioid abuse. Due to a lack of data, the projected frequency of bipolar disorder and schizophrenia is not clear, but there is an association and connection between increased substance use, bipolar disorder, and schizophrenia (Charlson et. al., 2014).

Access to Treatment

Low- and middle-income countries and especially sub-Saharan Africa suffer from a large treatment gap for mental illness. A significant amount of disease burden is due to mental illness, and approximately only 10% of individuals with mental illness are able to access treatment. This is due to structural inadequacies, lack of research, and policy restrictions. There is a dearth of empirical evidence on how to fill this gap. This is particularly true for severe mental health disorders such as psychosis. There are very limited numbers of mental health researchers, and this is a major component of the gap in treatment. There are new initiatives working to increase access to mental health treatment in sub-Saharan Africa. For example, the Partnership for Mental Health Development in Africa (PaM-D) has worked to connect diverse stakeholders, collaborate with colleagues in other nations, advance mental health research, and create infrastructure to improve mental health research in sub-Saharan Africa. This partnership has resulted in 60 published papers and 21 successful grant applications for progressing mental health treatment in sub-Saharan Africa. It is an effective and positive initiative that warrants more support and attention (Gureje et al, 2019).

Another useful initiative for developing the necessary infrastructure is the OneHealth tool. The OneHealth tool can be used to estimate resource needs, costs, and health impacts of increasing mental health services. The tool proved effective in understanding the cost of delivering interventions and treatment for psychosis, depression, and epilepsy in Ethiopia, India, Nepal, Uganda, Nigeria, and South Africa (Chisholm et al., 2017).

Another positive initiative is the Sub-Saharan Africa Regional Partnership for Mental Health Capacity Building (SHARP), which is located in Malawi and Tanzania. It was created to address deficiencies in treatment access. The goals of SHARP are (a) to build research skills for mental health among Malawian and Tanzania researchers, (b) to work to implement research findings into evidence-based mental health programs and large-scale practice, and (c) to increase conversations between stakeholders to increase mental health services in Malawi and Tanzania. SHARP is made up of five factors that include introductory and advanced short courses, dialogue, on-the-job training, pilot grants, and train-the-trainer courses (Akiba, et al., 2019).

Currently, there is poor access to mental health services in sub-Saharan Africa. The services that do exist are usually accessed by the most severely ill through inpatient urban facilities. Mental health care is only available outside of a hospital in 50% of African countries. There are unsustainable nongovernmental organizations that provide temporary mental health care in emergency and post-conflict situations. Yet, these services do not address chronic disease burden and disability. They address selective, acute care situations only. A new health model that works with primary care practitioners and community-based organizations for mental health could potentially make a positive impact in this regard and is needed to address current and future concerns (Charlson et. al, 2014).

Resiliency and Protective Factors

Historically, health and food have been equated with happiness and well-being in sub-Saharan Africa. Mental health and well-being were associated with physical health and adequate food. The relationship between mental disorders and mortality and morbidity has not been historically accepted or sufficiently acknowledged, and there is competition for funding for development initiatives. Strengthening the connection between mental health and public health is essential for growing awareness and understanding of its importance for overall public health and societal development (Jenkins et al., 2010).

According to the Afrobarometer, joblessness is considered the greatest issue. However, a pervasive and unusual level of optimism among youth in sub-Saharan Africa serves as a protective, resiliency factor. This optimism tends to decrease with age but serves as a strengthening, protective mechanism for mental health despite harsh circumstances or challenging sociodemographic conditions. Resilience, religiosity, and positivity serve as protective mechanisms for mental health and productivity. Nigeria, for example, demonstrates unusually high levels of optimism in contrast to world standards. On average, future life evaluations are much higher in Africa than present life evaluations. This optimism is believed to help individuals cope with and manage challenging life circumstances. Optimism refers to the belief that many things will improve regardless of current circumstances (Møller & Roberts, 2021).

The optimism identified in Africa may be abnormally high compared to world standards but represents a protective mechanism for challenging life circumstances, hopelessness, and depression. Also, research demonstrates a high level of acceptance, flexibility, and adaptability to everyday life and its problems beyond the norm worldwide. The Gallup-Kettering study reported that 90% of respondents wished to change many things to improve their lives. However, even when changes did not occur, the optimism remained that change would eventually happen. The common belief identified in this study is that individuals will be very happy with their life in the future even if they are not very happy at present (Helliwell et al., 2017; Møller et al., 2017).

Another component that supports mental health in sub-Saharan Africa is religion. A recent Pew study of religiosity in 30 countries found that religion is, on average, much more important in Africa than elsewhere. The association between religiosity and happiness seems to support the possibility that religion can increase well-being, happiness, and mental health levels and provide a sense of hope and security (Helliwell et al., 2017; Møller et al., 2017). A great majority of individuals in this region have a strong belief in Christianity or Islam. Certain studies estimate that at least 90% of individuals across 19 sub-Saharan African countries belong to Christian or Muslim groups. These beliefs are also integrated into traditional everyday cultural beliefs, rituals, and customs. Aside from this, there are pervasive levels of resilience through the practice of patience, acceptance, culturally embedded coping skills, and resourcefulness to combat pervasive mental health concerns (Møller & Roberts, 2021).

Another positive protective factor is the growing political and national interest in promoting mental health. There is a significant discrepancy in the quantity, quality, and impact of mental health in sub-Saharan Africa. The Africa Focus on Intervention Research for Mental Health (AFFIRM) project is an NIMH-funded initiative to improve capacity building for mental health research and services. AFFIRM provided research training for 25 mental health professionals, 90 researchers, and five Ph.D. students. The AFFIRM project is one of the first capacity-building initiatives for improving mental health in sub-Saharan Africa. More support is needed for this initiative, but it is significant as it supports the importance of a greater focus on mental health improvement in sub-Saharan Africa (Schneider et al., 2016).

Recent Changes in Mental Health in Sub-Saharan Africa

The world is experiencing a major health change as the aging population continues to rise and the disease burden is increasingly defined through disability and mental health concerns of depression, suicidal ideation, isolation, and loneliness. Health models predict that, in the next 40 years, sub-Saharan Africa will experience reduced mortality and a significant increase in chronic disease. Years Lived with Disability (YLD) estimates looking at mental health and substance use disorders from 2010 to 2050 were assessed using Global Disease Burden 2010 data and United Nations population forecasts. As a result, this significant population growth and aging will lead to an estimated 130% increase in disease burden for mental health and substance use disorders in sub-Saharan Africa by 2050 and an increase to 45 million YLD. Because of this, there will be a significant need to increase the mental health workforce by at least 216,600 full-time equivalent staff from 2010 to 2050. The anticipated increase in mental health and substance use disorders is predicted to significantly impact productivity and well-being in sub-Saharan Africa (Charlson, et al., 2014).

The COVID-19 pandemic has also created a significant rise in mental health concerns due to the actual experience of illness, social distancing and isolation, job loss, and feelings of stigma and discrimination related to the illness. Posttraumatic stress disorder, anxiety, depression, and insomnia have increased in sub-Saharan Africa and worldwide as a result of the pandemic. Training community health workers to provide mental health education, screening, and counseling services may be one avenue to help address these concerns. Toll-free mental health services and social media can be integrated to provide better mental health and psychosocial support services (Semo & Frissa, 2020).

The COVID-19 pandemic increased the incidence and prevalence of mental health issues in the sub-Saharan Africa region. COVID-19 created heightened levels of post-traumatic stress disorders, anxiety, depression, and insomnia particularly for women, children, youth, and the elderly. Social media and virtual mental health services have been provided to increase mental health education and communication services. Some interventions that can be provided, even post-COVID, include mental health and psychosocial support through mass media, community mental health education, toll-free mental health helplines, screening, and counseling services. From 2014 to 2016 West Africa experienced similar psychosocial impacts due to the Ebola virus including stress, grief, anxiety, depression, and PTSD. For example in Sierra Leone, a year into the Ebola virus epidemic, an estimated 48% experienced anxiety or depression, and 76% experienced PTSD symptoms. In addition to this, the utilization of mental health services is poor because usually services are used only when other social services and self-help mechanisms fail, and symptoms are very severe. Help is only sought out when symptoms are at a crisis level and very severe (Semo & Frissa, 2020).

A need exists to increase mental health and substance use disorder treatment. This represents a significant deviation away from the norm and current practices in a majority of African countries. There needs to be a substantial investment in training primary care practitioners, local community mental health initiatives, and growth in inpatient psychiatric units in district and regional general hospitals for these growing, unmet issues. Specifically, the number of people with schizophrenia, alcohol dependence, opioid dependence, bipolar disorder, conduct disorder, and major depressive disorder (MDD) is rising. The greatest burden for mental and substance use disorders since 2010 in the sub-Saharan Africa region is a major depressive disorder. It is expected to spike from 7 million YLD in 2010 to an estimated 17 million YLD in 2050. Although these estimates assume that current conditions remain constant, they are valuable for understanding emerging trends and societal conditions and concerns. The UN population data indicate that from 2010 to 2050 the population will double in size and the aging population will increase significantly. The data demonstrate a clear transition from communicable diseases characterized by high mortality to noncommunicable diseases that are disabling and chronic in nature (Charlson et al., 2014).

This rise in mental health and substance use disorders is significant beyond the quality-of-life concerns. It also has implications for economic impact and development. The cumulative worldwide impact of mental disorders is estimated to cause a loss of US$16 trillion in economic input over the next 20 years or an estimated 25% of the 2010 global GDP. Mental health and substance use disorders also increase the risk and prevalence of other noncommunicable diseases such as heart disease. Historically speaking, mental health has been low on the priority list for sub-Saharan Africa, and concerns such as malnutrition and communicable disease have been more at the forefront of concern. It is estimated that only 42.2% of countries in the WHO Africa region have a committed mental health policy, 67% of these countries have a mental health plan, and 44% have dedicated mental health legislation. In addition, African countries spend 1% or less of their health budget on mental health. Physical health is not separate from mental health. Malnutrition and communicable disease are strongly associated with major depressive disorder, and all of these issues are strongly associated with worsening developmental outcomes and increased poverty (Charlson et al., 2014).

However, there are barriers to drawing conclusions from the data provided. Out of the 48 countries in the sub-Saharan African region, only six had data to be used, which means a lack of information for the region. Other limitations included that protective and resilience factors for psychological disorders were not considered. Also, there could be bias in terms of the data that were able to be published and the data that have gone unpublished and unrecognized. Yet, in spite of these limitations, it is clear that mental health needs are a critical component of health care planning (Cortina et al., 2012).

LIST OF KEY TAKEAWAYS

- Mental health concerns are rising in importance throughout sub-Saharan Africa.
- The rapid growth of the population and the aging population exacerbates these issues as chronic diseases and illnesses such as mental illness and substance use disorder become more part of the norm.
- African optimism is a concept that is gaining significance in terms of resilience and coping, as well as the cultivation of hope for individuals suffering from lower levels of well-being.
- There is a major need to create mechanisms that address the current mental and substance health treatment gap as well as the anticipated future treatment gap.

REVIEW QUESTIONS

1. What surprised you about this chapter? How is the mental health situation overall in sub-Saharan Africa different from preconceived ideas you might have had before reading these materials?
2. What value do you believe the concept of "African optimism" could play in terms of an individual's perception of their happiness and well-being? How could this perspective be incorporated into other mental health initiatives?
3. What do you think could be contributing to the rapid population growth and demographic changes in Africa that are impacting mental health and substance use?
4. What are some unique protective factors that promote resiliency and positive mental health in Africa?

REFERENCES

Akiba, C. F., Go, V., Mwapasa, V., Hosseinipour, M., Gaynes, B. N., Amberbir, A., ... & Pence,B. W. (2019). The Sub-Saharan Africa Regional Partnership (SHARP) for Mental Health Capacity Building: A program protocol for building implementation science and mental health research and policymaking capacity in Malawi and Tanzania. *International Journal of Mental Health Systems, 13(1)*, 1–13. https://doi.org/10.1186/s13033-019-0327-2

Atilola, O. (2017). Child mental-health policy development in sub-Saharan Africa: Broadening the perspectives using Bronfenbrenner's ecological model. *Health Promotion International, 32(2)*, 380–391. https://doi.org/0.1093/heapro/dau065

Bauta, & Huang, K.-Y. (2021). Child maltreatment and mental health in sub-Saharan Africa In F. M. Ssewamala, O. S. Bahar, & M. M. McKay (Eds.), *Child behavioral health in sub-Saharan Africa* (pp. 67–92). Springer International Publishing. https://doi.org/10.1007/978-3-030-83707-5_4

Charlson, F. J., Diminic, S., Lund, C., Degenhardt, L., & Whiteford, H. A. (2014). Mental and substance use disorders in sub-Saharan Africa: Predictions of epidemiological changes and mental health workforce requirements for the next 40 years. *PloS One, 9(*10), e110208. https://doi.org/10.1371/journal.pone.0110208

Chisholm, D., Heslin, M., Docrat, S., Nanda, S., Shidhaye, R., Upadhaya, N., Jordans, M. Abdulmalik, J., Olayiwola, S., Gureje, O., Kizza, D., Mugisha, J. Kigozi, F. Hanlon, C. Adugna, M., Sanders, R., Pretorius, C., Thornicroft, G. & Lund, C. (2017). Scaling-up services for psychosis, depression and epilepsy in sub-Saharan Africa and South Asia: Development and application of a mental health systems planning tool (OneHealth). *Epidemiology and Psychiatric Sciences, 26(3)*, 234–244. https://doi.org/10.1017/S2045796016000408

Cortina, M. A., Sodha, A., Fazel, M., & Ramchandani, P. G. (2012). Prevalence of child mental health problems in sub-Saharan Africa: A systematic review. *Archives of Pediatrics & Adolescent Medicine, 166(3)*, 276–281. https://doi.org/10.1001/archpediatrics.2011.592

Glatzer, V. Camfield, L., Møller, V., & Rojas, M. (Eds.) (2015). *Global handbook of quality of life: Exploration of well-being of nations and continents.* Springer Netherlands. https://doi.org/10.1007/978-94-0179178-6

Gureje, O., Seedat, S., Kola, L., Appiah-Poku, J., Othieno, C., Harris, B., Makanjuola, V, Price, L. H., Ayinde, O. O., & Esan, O. (2019). Partnership for mental health development in sub-Saharan Africa (PaM-D): A collaborative initiative for research and capacity building. *Epidemiology and Psychiatric Sciences, 28(4)*, 389–396. https://doi.org/10.1017/S2045796018000707

Helliwell, J., Layard, R., & Sachs, J. (Eds.) (2017). *World happiness report 2017.* Sustainable Development Solutions Network. https://worldhappiness.report/ed/2017/

Ikwuka, U. (2021). *Living with mental Illness in a globalised world: Combating stigma and barriers to healthcare.* Routledge.

Jenkins, R., Kauye, F., Baingana, F., Kiima, D., Belkin, G., Mayeya, J., Borowitz, M., Mbatia, J., Daly, A., Tyson, S., Francis, P., Njenga, F., Friedman, J., Gureje, O., Garrison, P., & Sadiq, S. (2010). Mental health and the development agenda in sub-Saharan Africa. *Psychiatric Services, 61(3)*, 229–234. https://doi.org/10.1176/appi.ps.61.3.229

Møller, V., & Roberts, B. J. (2021). *Quality of life and human well-being in sub-Saharan Africa: Prospects for future happiness.* Springer.

Møller, V., Roberts, B. J., Tiliouine, H., & Loschky, J. (2017). Waiting for happiness in *Africa. In J. Helliwell, R. Layard, & J. Sachs (Eds.), World happiness report 2017* (pp. 84–120) . Sustainable Development Solutions Network. https://worldhappiness.report/ed/2017/

Schneider, M., Sorsdahl, K., Mayston, R., Ahrens, J., Chibanda, D., Fekadu, A., Hanlon, C., Holzer, S., Musisi, S., Ofori-Atta, A., Thornicroft, G., Prince, M., Alem, A., Susser, E., & Lund, C. (2016). Developing mental health research in sub-Saharan Africa: Capacity building in the AFFIRM project. *Global Mental Health, 3*, e33. https://doi.org/10.1017/gmh.2016.28

Semo, B. W., & Frissa, S. M. (2020). The mental health impact of the COVID-19 pandemic: Implications for sub-Saharan Africa. *Psychology Research and Behavior Management,*713–720. https://doi.org/10.2147/PRBM.S264286

Sequeira, M., Singh, S., Fernandes, L., Gaikwad, L., Gupta, D., Chibanda, D., & Nadkarni, A. (2022). Adolescent Health Series: The status of adolescent mental health research, practice and policy in sub-Saharan Africa: A narrative review. *Tropical Medicine & International Health, 27(*9), 758–766. https://doi.org/10.1111/tmi.13802

Ssewamala, F. M., Bahar, O. S., & McKay, M. M. (Eds.) (2022). *Child behavioral health in sub-Saharan Africa.* Springer International Publishing.

CHAPTER 6

MENTAL HEALTH AND HAPPINESS IN ASIA

"The first country to adopt happiness as an official goal of public policy is the tiny little country of Bhutan in Asia near China and India."
—Derek Bok

INTRODUCTION

This chapter discusses the topic of mental health and happiness in Asia. It first looks at the importance of mental health in Asia, followed by youth and well-being in Asia. Next it examines the positive strengths of mental health in Asia such as family, love, rituals, and spirituality. Then it explores challenges in mental health, such as the prevalence and after-effect of natural disasters as well as issues of cultural beliefs and mental health stigma that prevent treatment. Case studies of China and Bhutan are presented, and alternative supportive measures such as microfinance and mobile health initiatives are explored.

KEY TERMS AND DEFINITIONS

The following important terms will be introduced in this chapter.

Microfinance

- Microcredit or small loans are granted to individuals with low income.
- Microfinance assists in starting small businesses and can be accompanied by other supportive, empowering programs.
- Microfinance is an effective mechanism to support impoverished women, improve their level of physical and mental well-being, and provide low-interest rates with no collateral. Microfinance projects often provide savings, insurance, skills, and education training in addition to loans (Madhani et al., 2015).

REACH

- REACH refers to the response, early intervention, and assessment in community mental health (REACH) model to improve mental health.
- The REACH model was established in 2007 to help support school-aged children with mental health disorders.
- REACH is supportive of improving positive mental health and resilience in children by improving mental health literacy and providing a supportive environment for good mental health.
- The three main goals of REACH include improving (a) youth mental health through early assessment and intervention, (b) the ability of schools and community partners to respond to mental illness, and (c) the community mental health support network for children and adolescents in communities (Lim et al., 2017).

Mobile Health

- Mobile health (mHealth) refers to mobile technologies such as wireless mobile cellular technology that can be used for health and mental health initiatives and is a growing type of technology meant to improve access to resources, create greater awareness, and improve support for mental health treatment in the world.
- mHealth can help patients and providers to access health support in numerous formats such as text messages, calls, websites, and clinical decision support, to provide and receive health data, and to use health-focused applications such as certain apps or software (Brian & Ben-Zeev, 2014).

Gross National Happiness (GNH)

- Gross national happiness is a measurement of nine domains to assess growth, progress, and well-being first adopted by the country of Bhutan.
- These nine domains include psychological well-being, health, education, time use, cultural diversity and resilience, good governance, community vitality, ecological diversity, and resilience and living standards.
- The GNH index helps bring awareness and attention to the importance of mental health (Pelzang, 2012).

Overview

- Mental health is an important consideration throughout all of Asia.
- There is a paucity of evidence-based mental health interventions and treatments throughout Asia.
- A majority of mental health treatment is provided through mechanisms such as rituals, religion, spirituality, family love and support, public health education campaigns, and mobile health interventions.
- Interventions that address poverty and disasters are relevant for assisting in mental health improvement.

THE IMPORTANCE OF MENTAL HEALTH

Mental health is not a luxury. It is an essential part of functioning, quality of life, and overall health. There is a dearth of research on this topic in Asia. Some noteworthy studies include research conducted in Thailand and China. In Thailand, research on an empowerment program for HIV-positive mothers and, in China, a World Health Organization multisite study of suicide prevention are relevant. The research on the whole demonstrates a paucity of focus on mental health in Asia and an urgent need to promote mental health in low- and middle-income countries. The Global Action for Health Equity Network is one such measure for health promotion. Mental health promotion in low-income countries is a necessity and leads to improved mental health, increased health and social improvements, and strengthens individuals, families, and communities (Moeller-Saxone et al., 2015).

THE IMPORTANCE OF MENTAL HEALTH IN SOUTH ASIA

The definition of what constitutes South Asia is not completely clear. However, it is often considered to consist of Bangladesh, Bhutan, India, Nepal, Pakistan, and Sri Lanka. India, Pakistan, and Bangladesh are also deemed the most populated nations globally. South Asia comprises one fourth of the world's population and makes up some of the poorest groups in the world. According to the World Health Organization (WHO), health is a state of total physical, mental, and social well-being. It is not only the lack or absence of disease. Health, especially mental health, has been considered of low importance for policy makers in most of South Asia. Traditionally, in South Asia, families usually provide care for the mentally ill. If mental illness is very severe and beyond family care, the mentally ill may be locked or chained in their homes or abandoned. The structure for mental health treatment is extremely poor on the whole. The severely mentally ill often end up addicted to drugs, homeless, living in the streets, or infected with chronic disease (Trivedi & Tripathi, 2015).

The mental health resources that exist in South Asia tend to be located in urban areas and only accessible to a minority of individuals. Yet, on the whole, primary health care and mental health services can be combined together at a minimal cost to significantly increase the depth and range of service provision as well as address the treatment gap. It is important that sufficient political will and advocacy exists to bring awareness to these issues and implement practical, low-cost results. It is a human rights issue to ignore or avoid the impact and importance of mental health in South Asia and the need for treatment. A major contributor to poor mental health treatment access in South Asia is a lack of interest and commitment from governments. Cultural and political beliefs that mental health is not significant have negatively impacted the possibility of mental health treatment. However, on the whole, there is a growing movement and understanding that mental health is part of health in South Asia (Trivedi & Tripathi, 2015).

MENTAL HEALTH AND YOUTH IN ASIA

In the last decade, there has been a shift towards improving mental health services for youth in Asia. There has been a move from traditional clinic-based care to community-based mental health services. The response, early intervention, and assessment in community mental health (REACH) model is also an effective response to youth mental health in Singapore. It is estimated that at least 1 in 10 children suffer from mental health problems but fewer than one-third of these will seek help. Mental health disorders contribute to a major portion of the disease burden in youths. Poor levels of mental health negatively impact a young person's physical health, level of achievement, and social relationships, and increase their potential for stigma and discrimination. Poorer youth mental health levels are also associated with substance abuse, violence, suicide, self-harm, and accidents. All of these issues increase the healthcare burden (Lim et al., 2017).

Most recently in parts of Asia, there has been an active movement towards prevention, early identification, intervention, and mental health resilience for youths. Singapore is a small island state in Southeast Asia, and its need for outpatient child and adolescent psychiatric care has consistently increased. Community mental health centers have increasingly focused on providing services to children and adolescents. There is increasingly a shift towards more integrated community mental health care. In Singapore, the understanding is that many mental health disorders, such as anxiety and depressive disorders, begin in childhood and adolescence but are left untreated. Early identification, early intervention, and community-based interventions are needed in this case. For example, in Taiwan, an effective model is the "Taipei model" which includes community mental healthcare services in the primary and general healthcare systems. This model makes use of public health workers from 12 districts and provides follow-up visits to recently discharged patients. There is an emphasis on deinstitutionalizing mental healthcare and creating more community-based mental health services (Lim et al., 2017).

The REACH model was established in 2007 to help support school-aged children with mental health disorders. The three main goals of REACH include improving (a) youth mental health through early assessment and intervention, (b) the ability of schools and community partners to respond to mental illness, and (c) the community mental health support network for children and adolescents in communities. REACH is supportive of improving positive mental health and resilience in children by enhancing mental health literacy and providing a supportive environment for good mental health (Lim et al., 2017).

POSITIVE STRENGTHS OF MENTAL HEALTH IN ASIA: FAMILY, LOVE, AND MENTAL HEALTH

Positive strengths and inherent resiliencies that exist in Asia are also important to explore, identify, and investigate. Haliburton (2021) found that relative to developed countries, WHO data demonstrate that developing countries like India, for example, experience better recovery rates from severe mental illness than developed countries. This is believed to be due to the degree and quality of family support and the role of love in recovery. The degree, quality, and role of love in recovery in developed countries is much lower and poorer than it is in countries such as India and generally in Asia. India also has the best outcomes for severe mental illnesses such as schizophrenia due to positive family support and the experience of love, or what might be termed as unconditional positive regard. Another term for it is *sneham*, or caring love, which is a type of familial and friend love (Halliburton, 2021).

When individuals are hospitalized for severe mental illness, the family is very involved in visitation treatment in India, and this has been shown to generally have positive outcomes. Research from India suggests that the quality of an individual's family life and family member involvement directly and consistently impacts their degree of illness or recovery. The greater and the higher quality of family involvement and care, the better the recovery. The Movement for Global Mental Health has identified India as an environment of mental health deficiency and abuse. However, WHO data demonstrate some positive attributes that can be emulated and learned from. A case study of India illustrates both strengths and weaknesses in mental health treatment and care (Halliburton, 2021).

POSITIVE STRENGTHS OF MENTAL HEALTH IN ASIA: THE IMPORTANCE OF RITUAL

A kind of global mental health therapy that has existed throughout our known human history is the use of rituals. When individuals throughout the world experience extreme mental suffering they perform rituals. The use of ritual worldwide as a kind of global mental health therapy has been inadequately recognized by psychology and psychiatry. Religion and ritual have been used extensively throughout time and are very widespread throughout the world. Few studies exist, but the ones in India that do exist have found that approximately 80% of the population uses religious healers for the treatment of mental health problems (Sax, 2021).

However, the trend of using religious healers for psychiatric needs is also seen in the United States. In the United States, approximately 43% of individuals with anxiety and 53% with depression use religious healers and complementary or alternative medicine for treatment. A UK study found that 42% of Indians living in Britain sought healers before seeking mental health services. Ritual practices are often seen as nonmodern or nonscientific; however, their worldwide use points to their significance and further need for investigation. The definition of ritual is largely unclear but tends to refer to healing practices that are not part of modern, mainstream scientific mental health practice. Abundant evidence indicates that rituals heal. However, we lack sufficient evidence on how they heal (Sax, 2021).

CHALLENGES OF MENTAL HEALTH IN ASIA: NATURAL DISASTERS

Humanitarian crises and disasters significantly impact levels of mental health. Southeast Asia has experienced some of the most severe natural disasters in the past decade but has been very unrecognized in world literature regarding disaster mental health. In the last 20 years, approximately 200,000 people have been killed and more than 300,000 affected in Indonesia. Disasters are associated with higher levels of depression, mood disorders, and posttraumatic stress disorder (PTSD) symptoms. They are also connected with feelings of loss, helplessness, fatigue, and withdrawal. In addition, they create traumatic and complicated grief symptoms as well as exacerbate disorders such as substance use and depression. A study in the Philippines assessed the psychological impact of a typhoon and identified somatic body symptoms, and emotional symptoms such as anxiety, fear, anger, cognitive challenges, and behavioral issues. The psychological impacts of the disaster negatively impact the recovery of a community on many mental health levels. Another study of mental health consequences of disaster in Asia found PTSD symptoms in up to 60% of the population immediately post-disaster. These symptoms decreased to about 30% of the population having PTSD symptoms nine months post-disaster and 8% having symptoms two years post-disaster (Hechanova & Waelde, 2017).

These data demonstrate that PTSD symptoms impact a majority of the population immediately after post-disaster but steadily decrease over time. Issues such as displacement and homelessness also negatively impact PTSD symptoms immediately after post-disaster. Additional impacts of disasters in Southeast Asia and Asia overall pertain to general collectivistic cultural values. Hechanova and Waelde (2017) have suggested that trauma is commonly experienced interdependently because people are disturbed about their family and close groups in crisis instead of just themselves. Southeast Asian culture and Chinese cultures generally manage painful experiences by helping others, staying busy, and volunteering. Culturally appropriate modalities such as art and theater may be the most impactful for promoting positive mental health after a disaster. Art and theater may be supportive for assisting in emotional expression without crossing cultural restrictions in emotional expression (Hechanova & Waelde, 2017).

CHALLENGES OF MENTAL HEALTH IN ASIA: MENTAL HEALTH STIGMA

Other components that impact the use of mental health services include the cultural shame and stigma of mental health treatment. Interventions that improve social support and interdependent coping mechanisms are relevant for treatment in Asia. Spirituality and religion are culturally appropriate ways to address mental illness. Also, the use of practices such as yoga, meditation, and herbal plants are also relevant. Media, school, community-based, and family-based public health interventions have proved worthwhile for disseminating information on psychological first aid, resiliency, and mental health symptoms that can occur post-disaster. The dissemination of this information allows for some level of support regardless of stigma and cultural mental health preconceptions (Hechanova & Waelde, 2017).

CASE STUDY: MENTAL HEALTH AND TREATMENT IN CHINA

China is a case study of rapid development. In the last 25 years, China's real GDP per capita has multiplied more than 5 times. This is an unprecedented accomplishment in any country. The development was so significant that by 2012 close to every urban household had a color TV, air conditioning, washing machine, and refrigerator; close to 9 out of 10 in urban areas had a personal computer, and 1 in 5 had an automobile. These signifiers of development were lower in rural areas but still relatively common by 2012 (Easterlin et al., 2021; Knight, 2018).

China is a unique country given its communist economic make-up, especially in the 1990s. In the 1990s, China's urban labor market was described as a mini welfare state with its workers seen as having an iron rice bowl. Due to the economic and government structure, anxiety and worry for one's job situation, future, and family security were close to nonexistent. Furthermore, a vast majority of individuals employed in urban environments were employed by public organizations. Through this employment, they essentially experienced lifetime jobs, subsidized food, housing, health care, child care, pensions, and the guarantee of jobs for their children when they reached adulthood. China's well-being and life satisfaction levels were fairly high with a score of 7.29, which paralleled Russia's well-being and life satisfaction scores of 7.29. There was very little differentiation across mean values in well-being in China with a mean score exceeding 7.0 for education, work, and income. This means that the high overall life satisfaction and well-being score was not attributable to disproportionate outliers, but rather a good overview of the actual well-being of the whole population (Easterlin et al., 2021; Knight, 2018).

CHANGES IN HAPPINESS RANKINGS IN CHINA

China's 2012 ranking was 6.85 in well-being, which represents a significant drop in well-being from the 1990 value of 7.29. In addition, China dropped from 28*th* in the world to 50*th* in a 2012 poll of the subjective well-being of 100 countries. From 2013 to 2015, China dropped further to the position of 83*rd* out of 157 countries for subjective well-being, according to the Gallup World Poll Ladder of Life (Easterlin et al., 2021; Knight, 2018). The data from China are a sharp contrast to accepted beliefs that happiness is directly related to GDP and the concept that economic growth is directly related to increasing subjective well-being. The change in rankings from 1990 to 2015 clearly brings fundamental assumptions regarding happiness, well-being, and mental health into question. It demonstrates a contradiction, like in the United States, between well-being levels and GDP growth. The relationship is not direct and linear as has been commonly believed (Easterlin et al., 2021; Knight, 2018).

By conventional knowledge, the incredible increase in China's GDP since 1990 should have led to major growth and increases in status regarding subjective well-being, mental health, and happiness. However, four different surveys beginning in the 1990s indicate this is not the case. In fact, these four surveys all fail to demonstrate a direct relationship between increased happiness, well-being, and mental health with the increase in GDP. In contrast, all four surveys show significant declines in well-being since China's incredible GDP growth. Inflation was also assessed to look at the relationship between GDP growth and subjective well-being. Inflation increases, when accounted for, also did not impact the relationship between GDP growth and happiness (Easterlin et al., 2021; Knight, 2018).

Research into how China's change in subjective well-being compares to other regions with socialism also demonstrates similar effects. The European countries with subjective well-being data extending back to the socialist period also demonstrate similar declines in subjective well-being but lack a comparable GDP increase. Two components that seem to be important concerning subjective well-being in China include the issues of unemployment and the social safety net. The most significant component that can be pointed to is the change in unemployment rates from close to zero in the 1990s to double digits from 2000 to 2005, then declining moderately. From 1992 to 2004, 50 million people out of 78 million working in public organizations were laid off from work, and an additional 20 million lost their jobs in urban organizations. This job loss also led to a loss of public benefits and increased mental illness for those who remained employed but were afraid of eventually losing their jobs. In addition, the Chinese government implemented new policies that eradicated guaranteed employment and lifetime benefits. This is in juxtaposition with the growth rate of GDP, which was much higher in 2002 than in 2014. This experience in China demonstrates the significance of employment and its corresponding social safety net for mental health, well-being, and happiness. The decrease in these factors led to increases in mental illness and significant decreases in well-being (Easterlin et al., 2021; Knight, 2018).

Aside from the impact of employment and the decline of the social safety net, another component that severely impacted mental health, well-being, and happiness was the decrease in interpersonal trust that occurred as a result of the government social safety net policy changes and employee layoffs. Trust and confidence in the system in which a person functions are important components for mental health and well-being. Other assessments of happiness, mental health, and well-being have been somewhat surprising. A recent investigation on the impact of environmental pollution on happiness found no relationship between pollution and overall life satisfaction. However, it did have some short-term impact on daily mood. Also, rising housing prices since 2000 in China have been associated with the development of increased life satisfaction (Easterlin et al., 2021; Knight, 2018).

When the significance of unemployment and the social safety net on happiness was further investigated, it was found that these two factors are very important for personal happiness. Employment and a social safety net provide income security, family life, and a positive impact on the health of the self and family. In addition to this, these are items that individuals believe they have some control over and impact their day-to-day life. At present, subjective well-being has increased in China from its low in 1995 to 2005. However, this change has not been equal (Easterlin et al., 2021; Knight, 2018).

The data currently indicate greater equality and similarity in life satisfaction rates before the unemployment and social safety net changes than at present. Currently, life satisfaction is significantly different for the top third as compared to the bottom third regarding socioeconomic status. Individuals under age 30 have higher levels of well-being, which is reinforced by having a college education. Furthermore, subjective well-being has been greater in China's urban regions than in rural areas, which is a common trend in developing countries. These data come from the 1995 World Values Survey, the China General Social Surveys conducted annually since 2005, and the annual surveys since 2006 by the Gallup World Poll. It is important to note that China is a unique case study for mental health, well-being, and happiness. Few societies have experienced the level and depth of change in such a short amount of time that China has undergone. Repeated social transformation can be traumatic not only to individuals but to families, societies, and cultures. The negative change in subjective well-being demonstrates increased anxiety and stress over the new labor market (Easterlin et al., 2021; Knight, 2018).

CASE STUDY: MENTAL HEALTH IN BHUTAN

Bhutan is a small country in the eastern Himalayas. Limited reliable data on mental illness in Bhutan is available. From the data available on identified mental illness, an estimated 30% of those surveyed suffer from depression, 20% from anxiety, 10% from psychosis, 40% from alcohol/substance abuse disorders, and 30% from mood disorders (Pelzang, 2012). However, the data are from a limited sample size of individuals treated at the National Referral Hospital. It does not reflect the population at large, but rather the dearth of data on mental health in the nation as a whole. An initiative, the national mental health program (NMHP), was created in 1997 to provide access to mental healthcare by integrating it into general healthcare practice. This program aimed to incorporate mental health into primary healthcare and thereby create greater awareness of mental healthcare in the community. In Bhutan, attitudes towards mental illness are strongly impacted by traditional beliefs in spirituality and religious ideas. Alternative healing practices are often used and are most accessible and culturally accepted. Mental illness is a public health concern in Bhutan; however, the creation of the gross national happiness index helps bring awareness and attention to the importance of mental health. Bhutan suffers from prevalent mental health concerns but still makes gross national happiness a priority. Establishing it as a priority creates awareness and education of its significance (Pelzang, 2012).

MENTAL HEALTH INNOVATIONS: MOBILE HEALTH

There is a relative lack of resources to meet mental health needs in nearly all Asian countries. Specifically, there are deficits in funding, providers, facilities, medication availability, and research in the area of mental health. Mobile health is a growing type of technology meant to improve access to resources, create greater awareness, and improve support for mental health treatment in the world. Mobile health refers to mobile technologies such as wireless mobile cellular technology. It is the most rapidly saturated technology in history. Country income has not been a significant hindrance in the adoption of mobile technology in Asian countries. Many Asian countries have mobile device adoption rates that greatly exceed the population in those countries. This is the case when individuals have multiple subscriptions and multiple phones. In addition to this, data use has greatly increased throughout the world. Mobile technology may be an effective way to address this deficit as the infrastructure is already in place for access and availability. Mobile health is referred to as mHealth. It can help patients and providers to access health support in numerous formats such as text messages, calls, websites, and clinical decision support, to provide and receive health data, and to use health-focused applications such as certain apps or software (Brian & Ben-Zeev, 2014).

Governments worldwide and particularly in developing countries have been connecting to academics, nonprofit organizations, and telecommunication outlets on mHealth initiatives. Internet-based psychotherapeutic interventions, short message services such as text messaging, and tele-mental health treatments can be powerful ways to manage gaps in services. In Bangladesh, the Department of Health and Family Welfare implemented a large-scale public SMS messaging campaign. These intermittent text message campaigns were meant to distribute health and disease information. It provided a major boost for increasing general health literacy and awareness. This approach could be applied to mental health literacy to help the general public understand symptoms, conditions, and treatment. Improving mental health literacy has been shown to be effective for early prevention and intervention in mental illness. This mental health literacy can be accompanied by information to contact hotlines, locate treatment centers, and find relevant websites (Brian & Ben-Zeev, 2014).

Public stigma concerning mental health is a major barrier to help-seeking behavior. Suicide, a significant concern in many Asian countries, is also illegal in numerous Asian countries, and this creates a further deterrent for obtaining treatment. Mobile devices such as cellular phones and smartphones can provide support for at-risk individuals to bypass stigma and other culturally related barriers. A suicide prevention program was implemented in Sri Lanka to provide support through mobile phones to patients discharged from the hospital after attempting suicide. This program provided private suicide prevention resources and support post-discharge; However, this could also be provided to individuals in the early stages struggling with hopelessness and suicide. Other potential uses of mobile devices are scanning medications via bar codes to make sure medication is not counterfeit. It is estimated that 25% to 50% of medication in developing countries is counterfeit. This is harmful and problematic in addressing mental illness treatment (Brian & Ben-Zeev, 2014).

MENTAL HEALTH INNOVATIONS: MICROFINANCE IN ASIA

Another positive mental health initiative is work to promote microfinance. Microfinance provides financial services to women in lower socioeconomic circumstances in developing countries. Microfinance initiatives in South Asia have proven effective for not only economic advancement but also for improving women's mental health. A systematic review of 12 quantitative studies from South Asia assessed the impact of microfinance on women's mental health. These studies revealed that the length and level of involvement in microfinance activities made a positive impact on women's mental health. Economic empowerment is an essential part of addressing biopsychosocial needs and works to improve the well-being of women. Women still represent the largest group worldwide and in Asia suffering from mental illness and lower quality of life (Madhani et al., 2015).

Research from both developed and developing countries has found a very important relationship between poverty and worsened physical and mental health outcomes. Microfinance is a wonderful way to offer support for impoverished women, improve their level of physical and mental well-being, and provide low-interest rates with no collateral. Microfinance projects often provide savings, insurance, skills, and education training in addition to loans. More than half of the world's poor live in South Asia, and microfinance offers an important opportunity to counteract poor physical and mental health conditions of the most vulnerable. The research demonstrates that 80% of microfinance clients are female with the largest number of these in Asia. The evidence shows that women spend more of their income on households than men and, therefore, women's well-being and mental and physical health improvement has a multiplying effect and helps more than one person (Madhani et al., 2015).

Microfinance is associated with increased control of economic resources among lower socioeconomic class women, improved decision-making power, better self-esteem, lower stress levels, and decreased levels of intimate partner violence. However, this is also based on the success of microfinance loans as loan debt can increase conflict, violence, and stress in families that are already impoverished as well as worsen mental health. Here, the term mental health refers to an outcome that includes (a) improved psychosocial functioning (self-efficacy, autonomy, authority, decision making), (b) absence of emotional stress (anxiety, depression, posttraumatic stress disorder), and (c) decreased rates of every type of intimate partner violence (Madhani et al., 2015).

CONCLUSION

This chapter discusses multiple components of mental health and wellness in Asia. It explores its general significance as well as its importance for youth. Positive strengths such as the use of rituals, spirituality, and family love and support are discussed. Challenges such as cultural beliefs, mental health stigma, and the prevalence of natural disasters are also explored. Case studies of China and Bhutan are examined as well as innovative approaches to improving mental health such as mobile health and microfinance interventions. There are many aspects of mental health in Asia, which is a region comprised of great diversity and population. It is worthwhile to understand its resiliencies as well as its weaknesses to best create effective interventions going forward in the future.

LIST OF KEY TAKEAWAYS

- Mental health and happiness are important throughout all of Asia.
- Asia contains inherent resiliency measures through rituals, spirituality, and family support and caring as well as mobile health and microfinance initiatives.
- Bhutan is home to the creation and significance of the gross national happiness index.
- Both unique deficiencies and resiliencies in mental health and well-being can be seen throughout Asia.

REVIEW QUESTIONS

- What was interesting or surprising to you about this chapter?
- What are the unique characteristics of the case study of China?
- What is special about Bhutan regarding happiness and well-being?
- What is one innovative approach that has improved mental health in Asia?

REFERENCES

Brian, R. M., & Ben-Zeev, D. (2014). Mobile health (mHealth) for mental health in Asia: Objectives, strategies, and limitations. *Asian Journal of Psychiatry*, *10*, 96–100. https://doi.org/10.1016/j.ajp.2014.04.006

Easterlin, R. A., Wang, F., & Wang, S. (2021). Growth and happiness in China, 1990–2015. In L. Bruni, A. Smerilli, & D. De Rosa (Eds.), *A modern guide to the economics of happiness* (pp. 129–161). Edward Elgar Publishing.

Halliburton, M. (2021). The house of love and the mental hospital. In W. Sax & C. Long (Eds.), *The movement for global mental health: Critical views from South and Southeast Asia* (pp. 213–242). Amsterdam University Press. https://doi.org/10.1515/9789048550135-008

Hechanova, R. & Waelde, L. (2017). The influence of culture on disaster mental health and psychosocial support interventions in Southeast Asia. *Mental health, religion & culture*, *20*(1), 31–44. https://doi.org/10.1080/13674676.2017.1322048

Knight, J. (2018). Rural-urban migration and happiness in China. *In J. Helliwell, R. Layard, & J. Sachs (Eds.), World happiness report 2018* (pp. 67-88). Sustainable Development Solutions Network. https://worldhappiness.report/ed/2018/

Lim, C. G., Loh, H., Renjan, V., Tan, J., & Fung, D. (2017). Child community mental health services in Asia Pacific and Singapore's REACH Model. *Brain Sciences*, *7*(10), 126. https://doi.org/10.3390/brainsci7100126

Madhani, F. I., Tompkins, C., Jack, S. M., & Fisher, A. (2015). Participation in micro-finance programs and women's mental health in South Asia: A modified systematic review. *The Journal of Development Studies*, *51*(9), 1255–1270. https://doi.org/10.1080/00220388.2015.1036037

Moeller-Saxone, K., Davis, E., & Herrman, H. (2015). Promoting mental health in Asia-Pacific: Systematic review focusing on Thailand and China: Mental health promotion in Asia Pacific. *Asia-Pacific Psychiatry*, *7*(4), 355–365. https://doi.org/10.1111/appy.12200

Pelzang, R. (2012). Mental health care in Bhutan: Policy and issues. *WHO South-East Asia Journal of Public Health*, *1*(3), 339–346. https://apps.who.int/iris/handle/10665/329848

Sax, W. (2021). Global mental therapy. In W. Sax & C. Lang (Eds.), *The movement for global mental health: Critical views from South and Southeast Asia* (pp. 271–300). Amsterdam University Press. https://doi.org/10.1017/9789048550135.009

Trivedi, & Tripathi, A. (Eds.) (2015). *Mental health in South Asia: Ethics, resources, programs, and legislation*. Springer Netherlands. https://doi.org/10.1007/978-94-017 9017-8

MENTAL HEALTH IN THE UNITED STATES

"All men are created equal and have the right to life, liberty, and the pursuit of happiness."
—Thomas Jefferson

INTRODUCTION

This chapter discusses the topic of mental health and happiness in the United States. It first explores the importance of mental health in the United States and then the unique aspects of well-being. Some of the unique aspects of mental health in the United States include cultural dynamics regarding gun ownership, volunteering, a growing aging population, historically low birth rates, and a large mix of both legal and illegal immigrants in the population. Other aspects examined related to happiness in the United States include the significant factors in United States' happiness, the impact of the Great Recession and COVID-19 on well-being, and the American happiness paradox. Possible ways to improve well-being in the United States are explored as well as projections for the future based on current trends.

KEY TERMS AND DEFINITIONS

The following important terms will be introduced in this chapter.

The United States Happiness Paradox

- The phenomenon that in the United States, income per person has increased approximately three times since 1960, but average happiness and well-being levels have not increased during this time (Sachs, 2017; Sachs, 2018; Sachs, 2019).

DACA

- DACA refers to the Deferred Action for Childhood Arrivals and is a United States immigration policy.
- It allows certain illegal immigrants who arrived as children in the United States to receive a renewable 2-years deferred deportation and eligibility to apply for and receive a work permit (Rodriguez et al., 2021).

The Great Recession

- The Great Recession refers to a period of significant economic decline for countries globally and occurred from 2007 to 2009.
- The Great Recession began with the housing bubble burst from 2005 to 2012. Certain regions such as North America, Europe, and South America experienced the worst impacts (O'Connor, 2017).

Happiness Inequality

- Happiness inequality refers to how much individuals differ in their self-reported happiness levels or subjective well-being.
- There can be great variability between individuals and within groups and cultures (Alderson & Katz-Gerro, 2016).

Overview

- Mental health is an important consideration in the United States.
- The mental health issues in the United States are unique and different from other regions of the world.
- The American happiness paradox is a uniquely U.S. phenomenon.
- Volunteering is an interesting and distinctive aspect of well-being and happiness in the United States.
- The emphasis on income as the most important demarcation of well-being in the United States has proven faulty and inaccurate; deeper understanding is needed to fully encompass the complexity of American well-being.

MENTAL HEALTH IN THE UNITED STATES AND TREATMENT

Overview on U.S. Mental Health

According to the *State of Mental Health in America 2022* report, mental illness is a significant concern in the United States (Reinert et al., 2021). In addition, happiness and well-being levels in the United States have continued to decline in recent years. Specifically, close to 50 million adults or approximately 20% of U.S. adults experienced mental illness in 2019. Since 2011–2012, the number of adults who have reported serious suicidal ideation has increased every year in the United States. In 2021, 4.58% of adults had suffered from suicidal ideation and more than 15% of youth had experienced a major depressive episode in the last year.

Furthermore, there is a major gap in treatment in the United States. Specifically, 24.7% of adults with mental illness report an unmet need concerning treatment, which has not improved since 2011. However, despite this consistent gap in treatment over the last decade, issues regarding unmet needs and the treatment gap have not been sufficiently addressed in the United States. According to the *State of Mental Health* report, approximately 60% of youth with major depression do not receive treatment, and more than 50% of adults with a mental illness do not receive treatment (Reinert et al., 2021).

Throughout the United States the level of mental health care varies. Specifically, states such as New Jersey, Wisconsin, Massachusetts, Connecticut, and New York report lower rates of adult mental illness and higher access to care. States such as Alaska, Alabama, Utah, Oregon, Wyoming, and Colorado have a higher prevalence of mental illness and lower rates of access to care. Youth in the United States have a higher prevalence of mental illness and lower rates of access to care in states such as Alaska, New Mexico, Arkansas, Arizona, Idaho, and Nevada. In contrast, Pennsylvania, Maine, the District of Columbia, Vermont, and Massachusetts have some of the lowest levels of mental illness and higher rates of access to care for youth (Reinert et al., 2021). In terms of policy approaches it is helpful and necessary to look at the whole picture of what is occurring throughout the United States, and, to do that, it is important to understand individual states and their differences.

The United States Happiness Paradox

The United States represents a challenging contradiction. Similar to China where GDP has also risen, the GDP has not been associated with increases in overall well-being and positive mental health since 1960. The income per person has increased approximately three times since 1960, but average happiness and well-being levels have not increased. Most recently, since 2013, per capita GDP has continued to rise, but happiness levels are now falling, which contrasts with the conventionally held belief on the relationship between per capita GDP and mental health and well-being. The targeted focus in politics on economic growth excludes important factors in well-being that include issues of distrust, isolation, corruption, and growing inequality. The United States was ranked *3rd* among 23 Organization for Economic Co-operation and Development (OECD) countries in 2007 and fell to 19*th* of 34 OECD countries in 2016. From 2006 to 2016, the U.S. level of social support, the feeling of personal freedom, and the number of charitable donations all declined, while the perception of government and business corruption increased (Sachs, 2017; Sachs, 2018; Sachs, 2019).

These factors point to the reality that the falling happiness, mental health, and well-being levels in the United States are associated with a social, not an economic, crisis. Data comparing 2023 well-being levels to 2006 demonstrate a marked negative disparity. Repairing social norms and conditions back to 2006–2007 levels would most quickly and reliably create the gains in happiness needed to improve mental health and well-being. Data from the Cantril Ladder indicate that achieving a restoration of happiness and mental health levels to 2006–2007 levels would require a per capita GDP growth from $53,000 a year to at least $133,000, not accounting for inflation. A focus on improving social conditions would be more effective, less costly, and more rapid (Sachs, 2017; Sachs, 2018; Sachs, 2019).

The issues with social concerns are not insignificant. They are directly connected to increasing rates of drug addiction, suicide, and mental illness and decreases in social trust. At present, trust in the government is currently at its lowest level in modern history as is the perception of a rise in corruption. Income inequality is at its highest levels in U.S. history with the top 1% experiencing nearly all the gains from economic growth in the last few decades, and the lower 50% continues to fall. This points to an expanding lower class and a decreasing middle class. However, the decline in U.S. happiness levels is not only a social crisis, it is also a health crisis that is being shown in increased mortality rates. This increase in mortality rates is directly associated with drug and alcohol abuse and overdose, suicide, liver disease, and cirrhosis (Sachs, 2017; Sachs, 2018; Sachs, 2019).

United States and the Great Recession

The Great Recession refers to a period of significant economic decline for countries globally that occurred from 2007 to 2009. The Great Recession began with the housing bubble burst from 2005 to 2012 (O'Connor, 2017). Certain regions such as North America, Europe, and South America experienced the greatest impacts. The lowest levels of happiness in the United States since the 1970s happened in 2010 as a result of the Great Recession and a negative long-term downward trend in well-being that had been occurring over time. Immigrants, adults, and males experienced the worst impacts of the Great Recession due to significant income declines and increases in unemployment (O'Connor, 2017).

A study by Sameem and Buryi (2019) found that individuals living in states and regions with lower unemployment rates experienced higher levels of happiness and lower rates of suicide in the United States. Conversely, individuals experienced lower levels of happiness and higher rates of suicide in regions and states with higher levels of unemployment (Sameem & Buryi, 2019). Happiness has more recently come into the field of investigation regarding economics. According to research by Sameem and Buryi (2019), happiness depends on three sets of factors. First, personality factors such as age, gender, education, and health are very significant. Second, economic factors such as unemployment, income, and inflation are important. Third, political factors have a direct impact on happiness and well-being. Living in a state in the United States with higher unemployment actually increases the chances of committing suicide, according to Sameem and Buryi (2019). The policy implications of this are that the United States sees a higher probability of suicide cases during recessionary periods. Individual happiness from a policy perspective may actually also be a smart economic policy in the United States, as many policies that increase happiness are also good for the economy, such as improving employment rates (Sameem & Buryi, 2019).

Five Significant Factors in United States Happiness

One factor that significantly impacts American happiness is trust in government and income inequality. The substantial increase of mega-dollars in U.S. politics, with multibillion-dollar campaigns financing federal elections, political candidates, and corporate lobbyists, has had a negative impact on U.S. trust in politics. This has created a situation in which U.S. Americans do not believe politicians have U.S. interests at heart. Rather, the politicians work for the interest of powerful lobbies, other politicians, and wealthy Americans (Sachs, 2017; Sachs, 2018; Sachs, 2019).

A second factor negatively impacting U.S. well-being and mental illness is rising income and wealth inequality. Since the 1980s, there have been ongoing policies in the direction of protecting and helping the super-rich. This has created an ever-growing income gap with the ultra-wealthy having power and wealth over a majority of U.S. resources. A third factor that is significant is the decrease in social trust and increase of the Hispanic population. This relates to increased levels of segregation between diverse groups. A fourth factor is the dualism that was created as a result of the U.S. reaction to 9/11. The U.S. war on terror has created an "us versus them" mentality and unnecessarily increased U.S. levels of fear, terror, and anxiety (Sachs, 2017; Sachs, 2018; Sachs, 2019).

A fifth factor to consider is the alarming decline in the U.S. educational system. The cost of a college degree continues to increase, while the number of Americans completing a college degree is stagnant at 36%. Therefore, even though it is more necessary now than ever before to have a college degree to obtain sustainable employment, it is increasingly difficult and costly. This has also led to the US$1 trillion of student debt and countless youth with partially completed bachelor's degrees who have a challenging, uncertain future ahead of them (Sachs, 2017; Sachs, 2018; Sachs, 2019).

The United States and Social and Family Connections

Another unique component of well-being in the United States concerns the decline in social and family connections and the rise of loneliness and isolation. These include the upswing in addiction and the addiction crisis in the United States. There has been an ongoing crisis with heroin and methamphetamine use, and currently there is a growing fentanyl overdose crisis (Sachs, 2017; Sachs, 2018; Sachs, 2019). During the COVID pandemic, more U.S. Americans died every day from drug overdoses than from COVID-19. Addiction creates not only a potentially lethal crisis for the individual, but it also causes severe damage to families, relationships, and society as a whole. It leads to higher levels of crime, violence, and greater mistrust among people. It harms society on many levels and contributes to the overall decreasing levels of American happiness. The data show that improving and repairing social conditions is the most effective way to increase and improve U.S. levels of happiness. This may require changes in government policy and cultural values to successfully achieve (Sachs, 2017; Sachs, 2018; Sachs, 2019).

Happiness Inequality in the United States

In many ways, subjective well-being is established more through relative than absolute terms. Once a certain level of well-being is attained, happiness is often perceived in relation to one's culture, community, environment, and society. However, once basic needs are met, rises in average income do not necessarily increase rates of happiness. As income rises over time, our relevant standards shift and the new income eventually becomes normalized. At this point, people on average report they are not happier than before the income increase. Status is relative; income improvement is relative. After societies rise above absolute deprivation, factors of relativity become more significant. Certain factors such as marriage, health, social integration/support, and social trust are all important factors in sustainable well-being and happiness beyond income increases (Alderson & Katz-Gerro, 2016).

Data from the General Social Survey (N= 44,198) indicate a positive correlation between socioeconomic status and happiness from the 1970s to the 2010s. The association in this relationship was found to be linear, with a direct association between rising income and rising happiness levels. Since 2016, the United States has been experiencing a growing class divide, with the wealthy further increasing their income and low-income and middle-income individuals experiencing a greater decrease in income. In addition to this growing class divide, behavioral differences between higher-income, college-educated individuals and lower-income, less-educated individuals have increased (Twenge & Cooper, 2022). Lower-income individuals are less likely to marry or attend religious services. Both of these behaviors are positively associated with higher levels of happiness.

Another growing class divide is the difference between physical health, mortality, well-being, and individuals with 4-year college degrees. U.S. adults with higher levels of income, education, and status were found to be happier than lower socioeconomic status (SES) individuals in the United States. Overall, it is difficult to understand the growing class divide in well-being and happiness in the United States. But the data from the analysis of this survey suggest that the growing class divide in rates of marriage may be a significant variable. The data indicate that marriage exerts a positive influence on happiness. Some evidence has demonstrated that drugs, alcohol, and suicide have all played a major part in the growing class divide, not only in wealth but also in health, happiness, and relationships (Twenge & Cooper, 2022).

An analysis of how happiness has evolved over the period of 1972 to 2006 has found that no aggregate increase in happiness. However, happiness inequality has substantially decreased over this time. There have been significant improvements in the happiness gap from 1972 to 2006. Approximately two-thirds of the Black-White happiness gap has been eliminated, and the gender happiness gap is completely gone. Stevenson and Wolfers (2008) investigated why average levels of happiness have not grown in the United States despite continued economic growth. Generally, and historically, in the United States, those who are either wealthy, educated, White, married, or female tend to be happier than those who are either Black, uneducated, single, male, or low-income. This points to a significant happiness inequality gap within specific demographic groups (Stevenson & Wolfers, 2008).

UNIQUE ASPECTS OF HAPPINESS AND WELL-BEING IN THE UNITED STATES

Longevity and Happiness in the United States

Using the General Social Survey-National Death index dataset and Cox proportional-hazards model, Lawrence et al. (2015) discovered that overall happiness is related to longer lives lived among U.S. adults. Compared to "very happy people," the risk of death was 14% higher for those who "are not happy." The United States has in recent years, and for the first time. been witnessing a downward trend in longevity of both males and females (Lawrence et al., 2015). Factors such as happiness are relevant to explore to understand methods to improve longevity and quality of life. This is especially true as the nation continues to experiences a significantly growing elderly population and currently the lowest birth rate in the nation's history. A focus on the elderly populations is important as the United States understands the factors impacting mental health and happiness (Lawrence et al., 2015).

Volunteering and Happiness in the United States

Although income has been historically emphasized in happiness and well-being research, Gimenez-Nadal and Molina (2015) have shown that individuals who volunteer or do voluntary activities at any point in the day report higher levels of daily happiness than those who do not. Numerous activities were investigated, and the researchers found that volunteering was considered the most enjoyable and uplifting. The United States has a significant history in community service and volunteering and is a leader among western countries in this respect (Gimenez-Nadal & Molina, 2015).

For example, U.S. adults are two times more likely to do volunteer community work than either French or German adults. This participation in community activities has only increased over time. Volunteering increases subjective well-being, the experience of individual utility, and individual heterogeneity. Volunteering here refers to any activity in which time is freely given for the benefit of other individuals, groups, or organizations. It relates to the daily application of altruistic behavior in some form. In the United States, approximately 50% of adults do some form of volunteer work or altruistic behaviors regularly. This is estimated to be similar to the equivalent of 5 million jobs. Volunteering also seems to be associated with increased productivity in the workplace (Gimenez-Nadal & Molina, 2015).

Gun Ownership and Happiness in the United States

An unusual aspect of U.S. culture is the perspective on individual gun ownership. In many ways, it was part of the founding history of the United States that its people have a constitutional right regarding gun ownership. A quantitative investigation analyzed 27 years of national cross-sectional data from the General Social Survey (1973–2018) using logistic regression and found that gun ownership was unrelated to improved happiness. However, gun owners were more likely to be married, and the relationship between marriage and happiness created the appearance of guns increasing happiness. Yet, taking marriage out of consideration, individuals who owned guns demonstrated similar levels of happiness to individuals who did not own guns. These findings challenge assumptions on either side (gun ownership or non-gun ownership) that guns have an impact on happiness and well-being (Hill et al., 2020).

MENTAL HEALTH AND THE UNIVERSITY IN THE UNITED STATES

The United States has some of the greatest variety and number of university students of any country in the world. An extensive literature review of over 5,500 journal articles on mental health and university students from 1975 to 2020 reported that there has been consistent improvement in mental health and well-being among university students, especially since 2010. Also, this result was consistently found across a range of many journal articles. There is greater awareness now than ever of the importance of mental health and well-being among university students and within universities. Other topics of interest are issues such as abuse, substance use, stress, and managing life changes (Hernández-Torrano et al., 2020).

COVID AND WELL-BEING IN THE UNITED STATES

During the COVID-19 pandemic, there was a significant spike in worsening mental health and behaviors among adolescent populations. A survey conducted in the United States between January 2021 and June 2021 found that 37% of high school students experienced poor mental health during the pandemic, and 30% experienced poor mental health in the last month. Of significant concern, in 2020, 44% of high school students in the United States reported persistent feelings of sadness or hopelessness, 20% had seriously considered attempting suicide, and 9% had actually attempted suicide (Jones et al., 2022).

A buffering factor for poor mental health, depression, and hopelessness was having close relationships with others at school. Students who felt they had close relationships with others at school had significantly better mental health with lower levels of depression, suicidal ideation, and suicide attempts. This was true whether these relationships were connected virtually through the computer, telephone, or other devices or in person. The important variable was the feeling of connectedness with family, community, or others at school. This experience of connectedness was significant for cultivating positive mental health among high school-age students both during and after the COVID-19 pandemic. The pandemic had a significantly negative impact on the mental health and well-being of high school students. However, this impact has also clearly shown the importance of connectedness and feelings of closeness, either virtually or in person, for high school-age students and their mental health (Jones et al., 2022).

IMMIGRANT INEQUALITY

An important distinguishing characteristic of the United States is the influence of its immigrant population on mental health and collective well-being. In 2018, approximately 45 million U.S. residents were born in countries outside the United States. They comprise approximately 13% of the nation's total population. An estimated 51% of the immigrant population is from Latin America and the Caribbean, 31% from Asia, and the remaining from other countries. Another distinction in the population makeup is the considerable differentiation in legal status among immigrants. In 2017, an estimated three-quarters of the immigrant population in the United States were authorized, legal immigrants (Rodriguez et al., 2021). Approximately 10.5 million immigrants were classified as illegal. However, the real number could be even much higher because it is difficult to account for illegal immigrants and individuals with no formal records or identification.

A large literature review revealed an intersection between immigration and mental illness vulnerability. Specifically, factors such as experiences of war, violence, trauma, economic challenges, isolation and disconnection from family and social networks, racism, and discrimination were all concerns that negatively impacted mental health. In addition to this, fears of deportation created increased levels of anxiety among immigrants and their families (Rodriguez et al., 2021).

Immigrants from Asia, Latin America, and Africa all generally use mental health services at lower rates than nonimmigrants, despite an equal or greater need. This is particularly true of males, those lacking health insurance, and undocumented immigrants. Social support has been found to be particularly important for positive mental health, and those who need mental health support tend to go first for support from family, friends, or religion (Derr, 2016). Additional factors negatively impacting mental health among immigrant populations include challenges and barriers in accessing mental health services. Issues such as language barriers and culturally competent providers can be structural blocks in obtaining mental health care. In general, immigrants access mental health care services far less than nonimmigrants in the United States. Immigration policies also impact the health of immigrants (Rodriguez et al., 2021).

Specifically, anti-immigrant policies were associated with mental health concerns such as anxiety, depression, and post-traumatic stress disorder. Concerns about housing discrimination, employment discrimination, and fears of deportation all exacerbated mental health concerns, particularly for those of Latin American and Mexican descent. These findings pertained to both adult and children immigrants. However, efforts, such as the Deferred Action for Childhood Arrivals policy, had positive impacts on immigrant child and adolescent mental health. Other positive considerations include strengths-based approaches. For example, the national nonprofit *Welcoming America* promotes and supports positive interactions and outcomes for immigrant populations. Another positive, strengths-based program, *Adelante*, works to strengthen young immigrants through education on health promotion behaviors, strengths and resilience, improving community and peer networks, and improving employment opportunities (Rodriguez et al., 2021).

CONCLUSION

This chapter discusses multiple components of mental health and wellness in the United States. It explores its general significance as well as its importance for specific populations. These populations include immigrants, youth, the elderly, volunteers, gun owners, and other unique groups in the United States in relation to happiness and well-being. Solutions such as improving family and social relations are explored, and the American paradox is discussed.

LIST OF KEY TAKEAWAYS

- Mental health and happiness are important considerations throughout the United States.
- The United States is home to unique happiness variables
- Some unique components of the United States are its population of immigrants, the percentage of the population that owns guns, the percentage of the population that volunteer, and the heavy use of electronic devices and social media in the population
- The United States has demonstrated a policy emphasis on economic growth in relation to improving well-being standards.
- The American happiness paradox emphasizes the overall lack of happiness growth in spite of consistent economic growth over many decades.

REVIEW QUESTIONS

- What was surprising to you about this chapter?
- What components are contributing to the stalling and decline in U.S. happiness?
- What significance does the United States case study demonstrate regarding well-being? How is it unique from other regions of the world?
- How are the United States' changing demographics relevant regarding happiness and well-being in the future for policy?

REFERENCES

Alderson, A. S. & Katz-Gerro, T. (2016). Compared to whom? Inequality, social comparison, and happiness in the United States. *Social Forces, 95*(1), 25–53. https://doi.org/10.1093/sf/sow042

Derr, A. S. (2016). Mental health service use among immigrants in the United States: A systematic review. *Psychiatric Services, 67*(3), 265–274. https://doi.org/10.1176/appi.ps.201500004

Gimenez-Nadal, J. I., & Molina, J. A. (2015). Voluntary activities and daily happiness in the United States. *Economic Inquiry, 53*(4), 1735–1750. https://doi.org/10.1111/ecin.12227

Hernández-Torrano, D., Ibrayeva, L., Sparks, J., Lim, N., Clementi, A., Almukhambetova, A., Nurtayev, Y., & Muratkyzy, A. (2020). Mental health and well-being of university students: A bibliometric mapping of the literature. *Frontiers in Psychology, 11*, 1226. https://doi.org/10.3389/fpsyg.2020.01226

Hill, T. D., Dowd-Arrow, B., Davis, A. P., & Burdette, A. M. (2020). Happiness is a warm gun? Gun ownership and happiness in the United States (1973–2018). *SSM–Population Health, 10.* https://doi.org/10.1016/j.ssmph.2020.100536

Jones, S. E., Ethier, K. A., Hertz, M., DeGue, S., Le, V. D., Thornton, J., Lim, C., Dittus, P. J., & Geda, S. (2022). Mental health, suicidality, and connectedness among high school students during the COVID-19 pandemic—Adolescent behaviors and experiences survey, United States, January–June 2021. *Morbidity and Mortality Week Report, Supplements, 71*(3), 16–21. https://www.cdc.gov/mmwr/volumes/71/su/su7103a3.htm

Lawrence, E. M., Rogers, R. G., & Wadsworth, T. (2015). Happiness and longevity in the United States. *Social Science & Medicine, 145*, 115–119. https://doi.org/10.1016/j.socscimed.2015.09.020

O'Connor, K. J. (2017). Who suffered most from the great recession? Happiness in the United States. *RSF: The Russell Sage Foundation Journal of the Social Sciences, 3*(3), 72–99. https://doi.org/10.7758/rsf.2017.3.3.04

Reinert, M., Fritze, D., & Nguyen, T. (2021). *The state of mental health in America 2022.* Mental Health America. https://mhanational.org/sites/default/files/2022%20State%20of%20Mental%20Health%20in%20America.pdf

Rodriguez, D. X., Hill, J., & McDaniel, P. N. (2021). A scoping review of literature about mental health and well-being among immigrant communities in the United States. *Health Promotion Practice, 22*(2), 181–192. https://doi.org/10.1177/1524839920942511

Sachs, J. D. (2017). Restoring American happiness. *In J. Helliwell, R. Layard, & J. Sachs (Eds.), World happiness report 2017* (pp. 178–183. Sustainable Development Solutions Network. https://worldhappiness.report/ed/2017/

Sachs, J. D. (2018). America's health crisis and the Easterlin paradox. *In J. Helliwell, R. Layard, & J. Sachs (Eds.), World happiness report, 2018*, (pp. 146159). Sustainable Development Solutions Network. https://worldhappiness.report/ed/2018/

Sachs, J. D. (2019). Addiction and unhappiness in America. *In J. Helliwell, R. Layard, & J. Sachs (Eds.), World happiness report 2019* (pp. 122–131). Sustainable Development Solutions Network. https://worldhappiness.report/ed/2019/

Sameem, S., & Buryi, P. (2019). Impact of unemployment on happiness in the United States. *Applied Economics Letters, 26*(12), 1049–1052. https://doi.org/10.1080/13504851.2018.1529390

Stevenson, B., & Wolfers, J. (2008). Happiness inequality in the United States. *The Journal of Legal Studies, 37*(S2), S33–S79. https://doi.org/10.1086/592004

Twenge, J. M. (2019). The sad state of happiness in the United States and the role of digital media. *In J. Helliwell, R. Layard, & J. Sachs (Eds.), World happiness report 2019* (pp. 87–96). Sustainable Development Solutions Network. https://worldhappiness.report/ed/2019/

Twenge, J. M., & Cooper, A. B. (2022). The expanding class divide in happiness in the United States, 1972–2016. *Emotion, 22*(4), 701–713. https://doi.org/10.1037/emo0000774

CHAPTER 8

THE IMPACT OF THE GLOBAL TREATMENT GAP

"Human potential is the only limitless resource we have in this world."
—Carly Fiorina

INTRODUCTION

This chapter discusses the negative impacts that insufficient or inadequate recognition and treatment of mental illness have on societies around the world. Poor and inadequate mental health treatment has significant negative impacts on every country in the world, regardless of whether it is a "highly developed" country or an "underdeveloped" country. In every part of the world, mental health treatment is inadequate and does not meet the need. Only a difference in the level of unmet need and the variation in need exist. For example, the United States is experiencing an addiction and overdose epidemic and its accompanying co-occurring mental health concerns. However, the mental health issues in the United States are not the same as in India, for example, or Japan. There is both variation and unmet need everywhere.

KEY TERMS AND DEFINITIONS

The following important terms will be introduced in this chapter.

Mental Health Protective Factors

- These are characteristics that individuals, families, or societies have to help with managing mental health challenges.
- The factors may refer to inner resources, skills, strengths, practices, and coping mechanisms.

Overdose Epidemic

- Overdose deaths are the leading cause of injury-related death in the United States.
- The majority of these overdose deaths are due to opioids such as heroin and fentanyl, but more recently also due to stimulants such as cocaine and methamphetamine (Sachs, 2017; Sachs, 2018; Sachs, 2019).

Unconditional Positive Regard

- This refers to the fundamental acceptance and support of an individual regardless of what they say or do.
- This is a form of client-centered therapy and an important component of positive mental health (Halliburton, 2021).

Overview

- Mental health treatment is an important developmental concern.
- Cultures have inherent mental health protective strengths.
- Inadequate mental health treatment results in higher mortality rates, greater years of disability, more violence, poverty, chronic disease, addiction, and broken social relationships.

THE IMPACT OF MENTAL ILLNESS

Inadequacy of Mental Health Treatment

Mental health is at the forefront of concerns being addressed by WHO member states. As of 2020, 62% of WHO member states have been modernizing their mental health policy, and 40% have worked on revising mental health laws to better serve rising mental health issues (WHO, 2020). The amount of public expenditure that goes to mental health and the number of mental health workers is largely inadequate across the world. There are an estimated 72 mental health workers per 100,000 population in high-income countries and 1 mental health worker per 100,000 population in low-income countries. The global median number of mental health workers per 100,000 is 9, but there is major variation between low- and high-income countries for access to and type of treatment. In both high-income and low-income countries, mental health treatment is inadequately provided. Furthermore, more than 80% of mental health public expenditure is directed towards funding mental hospitals and not regular outpatient treatment or preventive measures. Mental health hospitals address the most acute, short-term mental health concerns and do not work in the community for prevention and treatment. A bulk of public health funding is directed toward mental health hospitals. This is a reactive, high-cost approach that increases the chance of disability due to mental illness. Hospital-focused, acute care, is inadequate at reducing mental health issues on a large, sustainable scale (Helliwell et al., 2018; WHO, 2020).

OVERVIEW OF PREVIOUS CHAPTERS

The previous chapters in this book discuss the unique mental health issues, concerns, and variations in the world. The discussion about the United States explores issues regarding addiction, depression, loneliness, and poor relationships as well as the overemphasis on income as a measure of well-being. The chapter on Europe discusses the issues of untreated and severe depression, the growing elderly population, and mental health stigma. The chapter on Asia examines the prevalence of culturally embedded approaches, family support, and ritual as well as the significant lack of inpatient hospital treatment and access for severe mental health. The chapter on sub-Saharan Africa discusses the rise of mental illness, the lack of mental health treatment, and the predicted rise of addiction and depression. The chapter on Latin America explores the importance of family and the ironic intersection between high levels of happiness, and positive, and significant relationships in spite of poverty and pervasive violence (Clark et al., 2017; Helliwell et al., 2017).

According to the World Health Organization (WHO), and looking large scale at all the regions, issues of depression and insufficient treatment exist in every part of the world. Currently, depression contributes to the highest number of disability days globally and is one of the biggest barriers to progress and development. It has a high cost on individuals, families, societies, and nations and means that individuals will most likely not reach their greatest potential for development. Ensuring that individuals, families, societies, and nations can reach their greatest potential has significant political, economic, health, and social implications (Clark et al., 2017; Helliwell et al., 2017; WHO, 2017).

Population Impact

Worldwide, the majority of individuals suffering from depression and anxiety include women, young people, and the elderly (WHO, 2017). Vulnerable groups tend to suffer from higher levels of mental illness. Depression is a major contributor to suicide. In 2015, close to 800,000 people died due to suicide, but a much greater number attempted suicide. However, due to the illegality of suicide and stigma, the number of individuals suffering from suicidal ideation and suicide attempt worldwide is still unknown. In 2015, suicide was in the top 20 causes of death, accounting for 1.5% of all deaths worldwide; it was the second leading cause of death among 15- to 29-year-old adolescents and adults. This is particularly significant in low- and middle-income countries where it is estimated that they experienced close to 80% of all suicides in 2015 (Clark et al., 2017; Helliwell et al., 2017; WHO, 2017).

However, since COVID-19, the pre-existing issue of depression and suicidal ideation has only worsened, and rates of mental illness are significantly higher today. Therefore, it is important to increase access to education and resources for depression, anxiety, and suicidal ideation, reduce stigma, and increase awareness of this global issue (Clark et al., 2017; Helliwell et al., 2017; WHO, 2017). The most effective approaches for societal change would include beginning psychoeducation in early adolescence so youth can learn tools to develop better understanding and management. Mental illness tends to worsen with time, especially depression and often begins in childhood and adolescence with little or no treatment (Clark et al., 2017; Helliwell et al., 2017; WHO, 2017).

THE RISING IMPORTANCE OF MENTAL HEALTH TREATMENT WORLDWIDE

Mental illness is a worldwide health phenomenon. The great majority of individuals with mental illness live in low- and middle-income regions of the world. The majority of these sufferers have anxiety and depression disorders (Helliwell & Wang, 2013; Layard et al., 2013). As of 2023, depression represents the greatest disability factor according to WHO. Those living with anxiety and depression experience 12 to 14 years of lived disability in Western, Eastern, and Central Europe alone (Helliwell & Wang, 2013; Layard et al., 2013).

A major issue in the global burden of mental disease is inadequate or absent mental health treatment, resulting in a major gap between need and availability. In 2013, the treatment gap for schizophrenia was approximately 32%. For more pervasive issues, such as anxiety, depression, and alcohol dependence, the treatment gap was more than 50%. A major treatment gap exists worldwide irrespective of the severity and prevalence of mental illness. This treatment gap has severe consequences for society. Mental health interventions are important for life expectancy, disability, and quality of life outcomes. As an example, admittance to the hospital for mental health reasons improves life expectancy by an estimated 15 to 20 years. Untreated mental illness creates significant problems for societies. Specifically, it results in major societal financial costs, strains healthcare systems, productivity loss, educational underachievement, higher violence levels, increased levels of addiction, crime, resource waste, social and familial decay, poorer physical health and greater obesity, and lower overall human and societal development (Helliwell & Wang, 2013; Layard et al., 2013).

However, despite its demonstrated significance for health, economic, and societal outcomes, no country in the world spends more than 15% of its health budget on mental healthcare. The outliers that spend close to 15% of their health budget on mental health include England and Wales. These countries have witnessed significant improvements in years and the cost of disability as a result of increased access to and use of mental health services (Helliwell & Wang, 2013; Layard et al., 2013). The cumulative effect of mental disorders is estimated to cause US$16 trillion in economic loss globally over the next two decades, or 25% of the 2010 global GDP. Low-cost, effective mental health treatments are available that can be made much more widely accessible and prevent this predicted economic loss (Charlson, et al., 2014).

THE IMPACT OF THE EUROPEAN TREATMENT GAP

Mental health problems are among the top public health issues in the WHO European Region. Approximately 35% of the European population suffers from mental illness, most often depression and anxiety. The number one chronic condition in Europe is depression, making up close to 14% of the total disease burden in 2015, with alcohol-related disorders comprising the second greatest disease burden. Mental disease disability accounts for some of the greatest proportion of social welfare benefits. Nine of the countries with the highest suicide rates in the world are in the European region (WHO, 2015).

One of the most pressing mental health issues in Europe is the growing concern about late-life depression. Horackova et al. (2019) found that 35% of the population in Southern Europe, 32% in Central and Eastern Europe, 26% in Western Europe, and 17% in Scandinavia suffer from late-life depression. In addition, this late-life depression heavily contributes to the total number of chronic diseases, pain, daily living mobility, strength, and cognitive limitation. There also is a 79% treatment gap for this population experiencing late-life depression. With a growing elderly population in Europe, this problem will only continue to have multiplying negative society-wide impacts without treatment (Horackova, et al., 2019). Late-life depression and depression in general in Europe have a strong association with chronic illness, diseases such as cancer, cardiovascular disease, cognitive impairment, smoking, alcohol abuse, and physical inactivity. This all creates higher years lived with disability and shortens average life spans as well as the quality of life lived (Horackova, et al., 2019).

One of the greatest issues for well-being in Europe is the treatment gap. Approximately only 20% of those needing mental health services actually receive some form of support. Treatment for mental illness has important implications worldwide for life expectancy, quality of life, and disability burden. Untreated mental illness creates major costs to society. It creates major financial loss but also strains healthcare systems. In addition to this, it results in lost productivity, educational underachievement, increased levels of violence, addiction, crime, less effective use of resources, breakdown of social and family relationships, deteriorating physical health and obesity, and lower overall human development. It holds society back from development; it does not help push it forward (Helliwell & Wang, 2013; Helliwell et al., 2013; Layard et al., 2013).

THE IMPACT OF THE AFRICAN TREATMENT GAP

The population of sub-Saharan Africa is expected to double in the next 40 years from .9 billion to 1.8 billion with a growing aging population than previously experienced. Population growth and aging will lead to an estimated 130% increase in the burden of mental health and substance use disorders by 2050 in sub-Saharan Africa. This predicted surge in mental illness and substance use disorders is projected to have significant negative impacts on health and productivity. The biggest projected concerns for the future are depression, alcohol, and opioid abuse (Charlson et. al., 2014).

Currently, there are very limited numbers of mental health researchers, and this is a major component of the treatment gap in sub-Saharan Africa (Chisholm et al., 2017). Health models predict that in the next 40 years, sub-Saharan Africa will experience reduced mortality and a significant increase in chronic disease. This is based on Global Disease Burden 2010 data and United Nations population forecasts. Significant population growth and aging will lead to an estimated 45 million years lived with a disability (YLD) by 2050 (Charlson et al., 2014). Specifically, schizophrenia, alcohol and opioid dependence, bipolar disorder, conduct disorder, and major depressive disorder (MDD) are predicted to increase. MDD is forecasted to be the greatest mental health concern and disability in the coming years and the greatest hindrance to health and development (Charlson et al., 2014).

THE IMPACT OF THE UNITED STATES TREATMENT GAP

As a global world economic and military leader, the treatment gap in mental health care negatively impacts not only the United States but other countries that could potentially benefit from its economy. The United States represents a challenging contradiction. The income per person has increased approximately three times since 1960, but average happiness and well-being have not increased. The United States was ranked *3rd* among 23 Organization for Economic Co-operation and Development (OECD) countries in 2007 and fell to *19th* of

34 OECD countries in 2016. From 2006 to 2016, social support, personal freedom, and charitable donations have all declined, and views of government and business corruption have increased (Sachs, 2017; Sachs, 2018; Sachs, 2019). Decreased happiness, mental health, and well-being levels in the United States bring attention to a social crisis. This social crisis is directly related to the rising levels of drug addiction and overdose, suicide, mental illness, and poor social trust. The social crisis is also associated with increased loneliness and isolation and the ongoing heroin and methamphetamine epidemic, as well as growing fentanyl use and overdose (Sachs, 2017; Sachs, 2018; Sachs, 2019). During the COVID-pandemic, more U.S. Americans died every day from drug overdoses than from COVID-19. Addiction also causes severe damage to families, relationships, and society as a whole. It creates higher levels of crime, violence, and greater mistrust among people (Sachs, 2017; Sachs, 2018; Sachs, 2019).

FACTORS THAT CREATE, MAINTAIN, OR GROW THE MENTAL HEALTH TREATMENT GAP

Mental Health Stigma

A significant impediment to effective mental health treatment is cultural and widespread mental health stigma (MHS). Stigma can create a sense of personal shame or negative identity, as a result of a person feeling that they are deviating from social norms. It has an important negative impact on mental health and prevents and deters individuals from seeking mental health care. Stigma is hypothesized to be as harmful to individuals and society as the experience of untreated mental illness itself (Bharadwaj et al., 2017). MHS is also significant in terms of the financial impact that untreated and pervasive mental illness has on society. It is predicted that the cost of mental illness is between US$60 billion and $300 billion annually in the United States alone. Aside from this, MHS and the associated lack of treatment negatively impact job productivity, unemployment, and job functioning. Individuals with mental illness are much more likely to be unemployed and underemployed than individuals without mental illness. In addition to this, at least 30% of individuals with severe mental illness encounter discrimination in both trying to obtain or maintain employment. Other forms of stigma associated with MHS include friend stigma, health insurance stigma, housing stigma, and family stigma (Sickel et al., 2014).

Mental Health Literacy

Mental health literacy (MHL) refers to knowledge about mental health disorders and their understanding, management, and prevention. As discussed in an earlier chapter, MHL is another important component of mental health and well-being treatment worldwide (Furnham & Swami, 2018). Health literacy is defined as "the ability to gain access to, understand, and use information in ways which promote and maintain good health" (Furnham & Swami, 2018, p.3). On a global and nationwide scale, the general public has a poor understanding of mental illness symptoms and is more accepting of self-help. This is in spite of the fact that WHO estimates that at least one-third of the population worldwide suffers from a mental illness. According to WHO, health literacy is a stronger predictor of health than factors such as education, income, employment, and ethnicity (Furnham & Swami, 2018).

Lack of Early Identification

Groups that are particularly vulnerable to developing mental illness are adolescents. Mental health disorders often appear visibly for the first time in adolescence and with young adults. Early recognition and treatment are critical for positive long-term outcomes, but professional treatment is not usually obtained or sought until symptoms have been severe. Early intervention will most likely occur only if children and their caregivers can identify early signs and indications of mental illness and access help. This is important for prevention and early intervention for youth struggling with mental illness (Kelly et al., 2007).

Lack of Political Will, Funding, and Focus

Despite its demonstrated significance for health, economic, and societal outcomes, no country in the world spends more than 15% of its health budget on mental healthcare. England and Wales have incorporated more government support for mental health interventions. There are low-cost and effective mental health treatments available that can be made much more widely available. It is illogical to not incorporate mental healthcare further into a country's budget when we see so many significant positive impacts on numerous quantifiers for development and wealth. However, at present, it is not largely of political importance for many nations, although WHO has made it a greater priority (Helliwell & Wang, 2013; Helliwell et al., 2013; Layard et al., 2013).

PRE-EXISTING PROTECTIVE FACTORS FOR MENTAL HEALTH

The Case of Latin America

The history of Latin America has created a general culture that emphasizes connection and interpersonal relations as a result of the mixing of native indigenous, Spanish, and Portuguese values. Overall, the Latin American culture values relationships as a central part of one's life purpose (Graham & Nikolova, 2018; Helliwell et al., 2018; Rojas, 2018). The family is a very important part of positive emotional development and purpose, and individuals generally live with families longer than in other parts of the world. Latin Americans tend to develop deeper relationships with those they grow up with and have long-lasting relationships. It is estimated that approximately one-third of adults still live with their parents in contrast to 12% in Western Europe and 9% in Anglo-Saxon countries (Graham & Nikolova, 2018; Helliwell et al., 2018; Rojas, 2018).

The Latin America data are important as they highlight otherwise overlooked variables for well-being, specifically concerning subjective, positive relational variables (Graham & Nikolova, 2018; Helliwell et al., 2018; Rojas, 2018). The positive affective state is particularly high in Latin American countries. This region generally ranks in the upper levels for well-being and happiness despite not being at the highest levels of income and other wealth factors such as education and employment. The research on Latin America highlights the importance of accounting for the affective state when assessing happiness. Latin American countries range from an average of 7.15 in Costa Rica to 4.93 in the Dominican Republic. The average ranking according to the

Gallup World Poll is 6.07. This is based on a scale of 1-10 for well-being with levels of 7 and higher indicating a state of thriving. Latin American levels of happiness are much higher than the average ranking in the world at 5.42. A unique case study within Latin America is Costa Rica with its very unusually high ranking of well-being at 7.15, higher than the average Western European country (Graham & Nikolova, 2018; Helliwell et al., 2018; Rojas, 2018).

From 2006 to 2016, eight of the top 10 countries for happiness worldwide were Latin American, and 10 out of the top 15 countries in the world for positive affect were Latin American. Some countries such as Bolivia, Peru, and Venezuela have higher levels of negative affect due to economic crisis, political polarization, high levels of violence, and family instability from migration and immigration. However, Latin American countries on the whole are outliers to what "should be" their levels of happiness when using common explanatory factors. The social organization provides a buffer to economic concerns and encourages and promotes increased happiness levels on the whole (Graham & Nikolova, 2018; Helliwell et al., 2018; Rojas, 2018).

One significant factor in the differentiation of Latin America in happiness and well-being is its focus on an abundance of family warmth and a wealth of supportive social relationships (Graham & Nikolova, 2018; Helliwell et al., 2018; Rojas, 2018). This is directly in line with the most recent well-being research that highlights the connection between relationships and individual happiness. Latin America in general has stronger social foundations and positive relationships in comparison to the rest of the world. There is a greater sense of relational purpose, which is associated with higher levels of happiness (Graham & Nikolova, 2018; Helliwell et al., 2018; Rojas, 2018).

The Case of Asia

The below section discusses aspects of well-being such as cultural protective factors, mobile health, family and relational support and the use of rituals.

Cultural Protective Factors

As discussed previously in an earlier chapter, Asia suffers from a significant mental health treatment gap like the rest of the world. However, Asia has an established history and overall cultural acceptance in most regions regarding spirituality and religion to address mental illness. Practices such as yoga, meditation, ayurveda, and the use of herbal plants are time-honored, culturally appropriate modalities to assist in mental health wellness. Other protective factors include the general cultural acceptance and inclusivity of technology and particularly mobile technology for the dissemination of mental health information needs (Hechanova & Waelde, 2017).

As discussed in an earlier chapter, in Indonesia, PTSD symptoms impact a majority of the population immediately after post disaster but steadily decrease over time. According to Engelbrecht and Jobson (2016), trauma is commonly experienced interdependently because of collectivistic values (Engelbrecht & Jobson, 2016). Southeast Asian culture and Chinese cultures generally manage painful experiences by helping others, staying busy, and volunteering. Culturally appropriate modalities such as art and theater may be the most impactful for promoting positive mental health after a disaster. Art and theater may be supportive for assisting in emotional expression without engaging in mental health stigma. Collectivistic cultural values play into the treatment and support of trauma recovery differently than in more individualistic societies (Hechanova & Waelde, 2017).

Mobile Health

Mobile health refers to mobile technologies such as wireless mobile cellular technology and is the most rapidly saturated technology in history. Income has not generally been a barrier to the use and adoption of mobile technology in Asia. Many Asian countries have mobile device rates that significantly exceed the population count. Mobile health is increasingly used to help support individuals in formats such as text messages, calls, and websites to provide and receive health data, and in the use of health-focused applications such as apps or software. Mobile technology can also help to overcome mental health stigma, mental health first aid, mental health literacy, and low political will concerns regarding mental health treatment (Brian & Ben-Zeev, 2014).

However, mobile technology can also be easily incorporated into government policy to provide low-cost, high-access, and impact solutions. In Bangladesh, for example, the Department of Health and Family Welfare implemented a large-scale public SMS messaging campaign to disseminate health and disease information. It increased general health literacy and awareness and could easily be applied to mental health concerns. Improving mental health literacy has been shown to be effective for early prevention and intervention in mental illness. This mental health literacy can be accompanied by information to contact hotlines, locate treatment centers, and relevant websites (Brian & Ben-Zeev, 2014).

Suicide is a major issue and also illegal in many Asian countries. Mobile devices such as cellular phones and smartphones are protective, positive factors to provide suicide prevention support without negatively engaging in cultural mental health stigma. As an example, a suicide prevention program was implemented in Sri Lanka to provide support through mobile phones to patients discharged from the hospital after attempting suicide. This program provided private suicide prevention resources and support post-discharge; however, this could also be provided to individuals in the early stages of struggling with hopelessness and suicide (Brian & Ben-Zeev, 2014).

Family and Relational Support

According to WHO, countries like India, for example, experience better recovery rates from severe mental illness than developed countries. Protective, positive factors such as family support and the role of love in recovery are cited as critical elements in this. Love, relationships, and family are not generally as involved in developed countries as compared to Asian countries. India has been found to have the best outcomes for severe mental illnesses such as schizophrenia due to positive family support and the experience of love, otherwise termed *unconditional positive regard*. Another term for it is *sneham*, or caring love, which is a type of familial and friend love (Halliburton, 2021).

In India, when individuals are hospitalized for severe mental illness, the family is very involved in visitation treatment. This has been shown to generally have positive outcomes. Data from India highlight how the quality of an individual's family life and family member involvement, directly and consistently, impacts their degree of illness or recovery. The greater and the higher quality of family involvement and care, the better the recovery. A case study of India demonstrates both strengths and weaknesses in mental health treatment and care (Halliburton, 2021).

The Use of Ritual

A kind of global mental health therapy that has existed throughout our known human history is the use of rituals. When individuals throughout the world experience extreme mental suffering they perform rituals. The use of ritual worldwide as a kind of global mental health therapy has been inadequately recognized by psychology and psychiatry. Religion and ritual have been used extensively throughout time and are very widespread throughout the world. Few studies exist, but the ones in India that do exist have found that approximately 80% of the population uses religious healers for the treatment of mental health problems (Sax, 2021). Ritual practices are often seen as nonmodern or nonscientific. However, their worldwide use points to their significance and relevancy. The definition of ritual is largely unclear but tends to refer to healing practices that are not part of modern, mainstream scientific mental health practice. Abundant evidence indicates that rituals heal, but we still lack sufficient evidence on how they heal (Sax, 2021).

The Case of The United States

Volunteering

Individuals who volunteer or do voluntary activities report higher levels of daily happiness. Volunteering increases subjective well-being, the feeling of individual utility, and individual heterogeneity. Volunteering refers to any activity in which time is given for the benefit of others and involves the daily application of altruistic behavior. The United States has a unique history in community service and volunteering and is a leader among Western countries (Gimenez-Nadal & Molina, 2015). Even with its current social decline, U.S. adults are two times more likely to do volunteer community work than either French or German adults and approximately 50% of adults do some form of volunteer work or altruistic behavior regularly. This is estimated to be similar to the equivalent of 5 million jobs (Gimenez-Nadal & Molina, 2015).

CONCLUSION

This chapter discusses multiple components of the mental health treatment gap that exists globally. It explores barriers in mental health treatment, the impact that inadequate treatment has on societies, and the importance of addressing the treatment gap. Protective mental health factors are reviewed as well as inherent strengths and coping mechanisms that exist in spite of treatment gaps.

LIST OF KEY TAKEAWAYS

- Mental health and happiness are important considerations, and there is a global unmet need.
- Factors such as volunteering, rituals, mobile health, spirituality, community support, and cultural practices provide mental health protection amidst the global mental health treatment gap.
- Concerns such as suicide, depression, chronic disease, broken social relationships, and addiction result when adequate mental health treatment is not accessible.
- Low-cost, high-impact interventions exist that can be implemented on a large scale to make a positive impact throughout many societies globally.

REVIEW QUESTIONS

- What was surprising to you about this chapter?
- What are already existing protective mental health factors in Asia?
- What are already existing protective mental health factors in the United States?
- What are already existing protective mental health factors in Latin America?
- In 2 to 3 sentences, discuss the ways that inadequate mental health treatment negatively impacts society.

ARY

Cont

REFERENCES

Bharadwaj, P., Pai, M. M., & Suziedelyte, A. (2017). Mental health stigma. *Economics Letters*, *159*, 57–60. https://doi.org/10.1016/j.econlet.2017.06.028

Brian, R. M., & Ben-Zeev, D. (2014). Mobile health (mHealth) for mental health in Asia: Objectives, strategies, and limitations. *Asian Journal of Psychiatry*, *10*, 96–100. https://doi.org/10.1016/j.ajp.2014.04.006

Charlson, F. J., Diminic, S., Lund, C., Degenhardt, L., & Whiteford, H. A. (2014). Mental and substance use disorders in sub-Saharan Africa: Predictions of epidemiological changes and mental health workforce requirements for the next 40 years. *PloS One, 9*(10), e110208. https://doi.org/10.1371/journal.pone.0110208

Chisholm, D., Heslin, M., Docrat, S., Nanda, S., Shidhaye, R., Upadhaya, N., ... & Lund, C. (2017). Scaling-up services for psychosis, depression and epilepsy in sub-Saharan Africa and South Asia: Development and application of a mental health systems planning tool (OneHealth). *Epidemiology and Psychiatric Sciences, 26*(3), 234–244. https://doi.org/10.1017/S2045796016000408

Clark, A., Fleche, S., Layard, R., Powdthavee, N., & Ward, G. (2017). The key determinants of happiness and misery. In J. F Helliwell, H. Huang, & S. Wang (Eds.), *World happiness report,* (pp. *122-143) Sustainable Development Solutions Network.* https://s3.amazonaws.com/happiness-report/2017/HR17.pdf

Engelbrecht, A., & Jobson, L. (2016). Exploring trauma-associated appraisals in trauma survivors from collectivistic cultures. *SpringerPlus*, *5*(1), 1-11.

Furnham, A., & Swami, V. (2018). Mental health literacy: A review of what it is and why it matters. *International Perspectives in Psychology: Research, Practice, Consultation*, *7*(4), 240–257. https://doi.org/10.1037/ipp0000094

Gimenez-Nadal, J. I., & Molina, J. A. (2015). Voluntary activities and daily happiness in the United States. *Economic Inquiry*, *53*(4), 1735–1750. https://doi.org/10.1111/ecin.12227

Graham, C., & Nikolova, M. (2018). Happiness and international migration in Latin America. In J. F. Helliwell, R. Layard, & J. Sachs (Eds.), *World happiness report 2018* (pp. 88–114). Sustainable Development Solutions Network. https://worldhappiness.report/ed/2018/

Halliburton, M. (2021). The house of love and the mental hospital. In W. Sax & C. Long (Eds.), *The movement for global mental health: Critical views from South and Southeast Asia* (pp. 213–242). Amsterdam University Press. https://doi.org/10.1515/9789048550135-008

Hechanova, R., & Waelde, L. (2017). The influence of culture on disaster mental health and psychosocial support interventions in Southeast Asia. *Mental health, religion & culture*, *20*(1), 31–44. https://doi.org/10.1080/13674676.2017.1322048

Helliwell, J. F., Huang, H., & Wang, S. (2017). The social foundations of world happiness. In J. F Helliwell, H. Huang, & S. Wang (Eds.), *World happiness report,* (pp. *8–47) Sustainable Development Solutions Network. https://s3.amazonaws.com/happiness-report/2017/HR17.pdf*

Helliwell, J. F., Layard, R., & Sachs, J. (Eds.) (2013). *World happiness report 2013.* Sustainable Development Solutions Network. *https://worldhappiness.report/ed/2013/*

Helliwell, J. F., Layard, R., & Sachs, J. (Eds.) (2018). *World happiness report 2018,* Sustainable Development Solutions Network. https://worldhappiness.report/ed/2018/

Helliwell, J. F., & Wang, S. (2013). World happiness: Trends, explanations and distribution. In J. Helliwell, R. Layard, & J. Sachs (Eds.), *World happiness report 2013. Sustainable Development Solutions Network. https://worldhappiness.report/ed/2013/*

Horackova, K., Kopecek, M., Machů, V., Kagstrom, A., Aarsland, D., Motlova, L. B., & Cermakova, P. (2019). Prevalence of late-life depression and gap in mental health service use across European regions. *European Psychiatry, 57*, 19–25. https://doi.org/10.1016/j.eurpsy.2018.12.002

Kelly, C. M., Jorm, A. F., & Wright, A. (2007). Improving mental health literacy as a strategy to facilitate early intervention for mental disorders. *Medical Journal of Australia*, *187*(S7), S26–S30. https://doi.org/10.5694/j.1326-5377.2007.tb01332.x

Layard, R., Chisholm, D., Patel, V., & Saxena, S. (2013). Mental illness and unhappiness. (Discussion Paper No. 1239) Center for Economic Performance, London School of Economics and Political Science. https://cep.lse.ac.uk/pubs/download/dp1239.pdf

Rojas, M. (2018). Happiness in Latin America has social foundations. In J. F. Helliwell, R. Layard, & J. Sachs (Eds.), *World happiness report 2018 (pp.* 89–114). Sustainable Development Solutions Network. https://worldhappiness.report/ed/2018/

Sachs, J. D. (2017). Restoring American happiness. *In J. Helliwell, R. Layard, & J. Sachs (Eds.), World happiness report 2017* (pp. 178–183. Sustainable Development Solutions Network. https://worldhappiness.report/ed/2017/

Sachs, J. D. (2018). America's health crisis and the Easterlin paradox. *In J. Helliwell, R. Layard, & J. Sachs (Eds.), World happiness report, 2018,* (pp. 146159). Sustainable Development Solutions Network. https://worldhappiness.report/ed/2018/

Sachs, J. D. (2019). Addiction and unhappiness in America. *In J. Helliwell, R. Layard, & J. Sachs (Eds.), World happiness report 2019* (pp. 122–131). Sustainable Development Solutions Network. https://worldhappiness.report/ed/2019/

Sax, W. (2021). Global mental therapy. In W. Sax & C. Lang (Eds.), *The movement for global mental health: Critical views from South and Southeast Asia* (pp. 271–300). Amsterdam University Press. https://doi.org/10.1017/9789048550135.009

Sickel, A. E., Seacat, J. D., & Nabors, N. A. (2014). Mental health stigma update: A review of consequences. *Advances in Mental Health*, *12*(3), 202–215. https://doi.org/10.1080/18374905.2014.11081898

World Health Organization. (2015). *The European mental health action plan 2013–2020*. World Health Organization. Regional Office for Europe. https://apps.who.int/iris/handle/10665/175672

CHAPTER 9

THE FUTURE OF MENTAL HEALTH TREATMENT

"Being able to be your true self is one of the strongest components of good mental health."
—Lauren Fogel Mersy

"Over the course of the past decade, there's been increased willingness to recognize mental health as an essential part of one's well-being."
— Nicole Spector

INTRODUCTION

This chapter explores the future of mental health treatment and what it might look like going forward. Currently, an epidemic of depression, suicidal ideation, loneliness, and isolation is growing worldwide. Mental health interventions and treatment will be increasingly needed as the world shifts and our concerns regarding these issues rise. These concerns are also associated with heightened physical disease, chronic disease, addiction, obesity, and societal and family deterioration. The future of mental health treatment benefits from assessing the larger picture of what is occurring in regions, countries, and within population groups and creating interventions that are appropriate for those groups.

The future of mental health treatment also likely includes larger-scale public health and social media campaigns to decrease the amount of mental health stigma, increase mental health first aid, increase the number of trained mental health professionals, and implement greater mental health services within the already existing health structures of countries. The future of mental health in many regions will also likely include a greater understanding of and knowledge about treating personality disorders, trauma, addiction, and psychosis.

KEY TERMS AND DEFINITIONS

The following important terms will be introduced in this chapter.

Solution-Focused Therapy

- A strength-based, trauma therapy approach that can be adapted for psychoeducation and offers effective, brief therapy interventions.
- Solution-Focused Therapy can be applied to support large-scale interventions and focuses on the strengths individuals already possess.
- It also focuses on the belief that people already have the resources they need to solve their own problems (De Shazer et al., 2021).

E-health

- Mental health interventions are applied through the internet, mobile devices, or other web-based technology.
- Internet-based interventions used for the prevention and management of mental illness, are readily accessible and are rapidly growing (Jiménez-Molina et al., 2019).

Public Health Campaigns

- Large-scale health awareness efforts through various mediums and forms of communication to communicate mental health literacy needs.
- Public health campaigns on mental health awareness, identification, and psychoeducation are important for the future to decrease the burden of mental illness in a low-cost, high-impact way (Sickel et al., 2014).

Overview

- According to WHO, mental health issues of depression and suicidality are among the greatest worldwide health issues.
- The factors of mental health stigma, mental health literacy, and prevention are crucial for addressing this current and future concern.
- Many low-cost, high-impact intervention options already exist that can be applied on small and large scales.
- The future of mental health treatment could lend itself to a greater normalization, integration, and widespread adoption of mental health interventions and improvement or to worsening levels if global need remains unmet.

MENTAL HEALTH PROGRESS

The field of mental healthcare has progressed significantly since the 1950s with new medications to help with depression, anxiety, bipolar, and psychotic disorders. In the 1970s, new evidenced-based therapy interventions were created including cognitive behavior therapy (CBT) (Helliwell & Wang, 2013; Layard et al., 2013). Treatment with CBT and medication provides recovery rates of more than 50% for anxiety disorders. Therapy and drug interventions are inexpensive, and there is no downside to increasing and expanding access to mental health treatment. Reducing the level of disability, addiction, obesity, crime, relationship deterioration, unemployment, and violence, eventually adds up to increased wealth and development in any nation (Helliwell & Wang, 2013; Layard et al., 2013).

The recognition of the importance of mental health treatment and the overall positive impact it will have not only on society, but on economics, led the British government to begin a therapy program in 2008 to increase access to services. This program is called Improving Access to Psychological Therapies (IAPT) (Helliwell et al., 2013). As of 2013, the program has served more than half a million people a year and continues to expand. The outcomes and rates of recovery are similar to clinical trials and have resulted in higher levels of employment and fewer years lived of disability (Helliwell & Wang, 2013; Layard et al., 2013).

The success of Britain's government-backed therapy initiative, IAPT, helped Chile to consider implementing a similar program. In Chile, research on the cost and impact of depression treatment led to its incorporation and prioritization in the national health care program. Depression is now considered a significant health problem in Chile even though in the past it was not. Two separate studies investigated the impact of increased mental healthcare in India and Southeast Asia and found that depression treatment created a minimum of 20 disability-free days. In addition, providing a minimum of 10 CBT sessions significantly increased individual productivity (Helliwell & Wang, 2013; Layard et al., 2013).

THE FUTURE AND CHILD MENTAL HEALTH

The future of mental health would be greatly served through widespread child therapy, youth psychoeducation, and prevention interventions. At least 50% of child mental illness is expressed by age 15. Mental health disorders often appear visibly for the first time in adolescence and in young adults. Early recognition and treatment are critical for better long-term outcomes. Child mental illness is often expressed through internalizing disorders, such as anxiety and depression, and externalizing disorders, such as conduct disorder, attention-deficit hyperactivity disorder (ADHD), and behavior issues. Child anxiety has a 50% to 60% recovery rate with mental health therapy, and depression has high success rates with CBT, interpersonal therapy, and medication. Mild to moderate conduct disorder, when accompanied by parent training, is treatable. ADHD has a 70% recovery rate with the psychostimulant medication Methylphenidate. The data clearly demonstrate that early intervention with children is very effective, economically sound, and preventive, so the symptoms do not worsen into adulthood. Early intervention programs and mental health initiatives serve as protective or preventive factors in mental illness (Helliwell et al., 2015; Layard & Hagell, 2015).

Intervention Approach

Interventions that are implemented in home, work, community, and school-based environments are effective for addressing youth mental health needs. Psychoeducational programs conducted by community members can provide effective, low-cost interventions for pregnant mothers and parents with young children. Psychosocial support through education and public health measures may be effective for addressing variables that put an individual at risk for developing a mental illness or for learning how to manage early symptoms (Helliwell et al., 2015; Layard & Hagell, 2015). Different types of interventions can improve mental health literacy and stigma, such as community, youth, school-based, and train-the-trainer campaigns. These kinds of campaigns can improve prevention and early intervention for youth struggling with mental illness (Kelly et al., 2007).

Treatment for mental health, as evidenced by the data, is as important as physical health, and children with anxiety and depression disorders are one of the most overlooked groups. Left without treatment, these conditions develop further and lead to higher levels of disability, greater treatment difficulty, and societal issues when these children become adults (Helliwell et al., 2015; Layard & Hagell, 2015). Some ways to further address these concerns are by training primary healthcare providers to be better able to identify and treat mental illness. In 2013, the World Health Assembly adopted WHO's Comprehensive Mental Health Action Plan to signify a political commitment for countries worldwide to improve mental health. The future of mental health will be more positive if there is a political commitment to improve health. Otherwise, there is a likelihood that the problems of depression, suicidal ideation, and mental illness will continue to rise worldwide as has been the trend (Helliwell et al., 2015; Layard & Hagell, 2015).

Overcoming Mental Health Stigma

Stigma has an important negative impact on mental health awareness, prevention, and treatment. Stigma is hypothesized to be as harmful to individuals and society as the experience of untreated mental illness itself (Bharadwaj et al., 2017). Mental health literacy is another important component of mental health and well-being treatment worldwide and an effective way to overcome mental health stigma. The general public has a poor understanding of mental illness symptoms and is more accepting of self-help approaches over traditional medical treatment (Furnham & Swami, 2018). Public health campaigns on mental health awareness, identification, and psychoeducation are important for the future to decrease the burden of mental illness in a low-cost, high-impact way (Sickel et al., 2014). Other significant mechanisms to improve mental health literacy include awareness campaigns, educational workshops, training courses, and mental health first aid training (Ganasen et al., 2008).

EFFECTIVE INTERVENTIONS FOR THE FUTURE OF MENTAL HEALTH

Mental Health First Aid

To address the enormous gap in mental health treatment worldwide in the future, aside from improving mental health literacy and decreasing mental health stigma, it is also important and effective to implement large-scale mental health first aid (MHFA) training. MHFA training teaches others ways to provide early help for someone who is developing a mental health problem or is in a crisis state. MHFA training can be provided through e-learning to educate participants about mental health disorders, stigmatizing attitudes, and helping behaviors. MHFA training has been shown through both e-learning and printed materials to increase knowledge, reduce stigma, and improve self-confidence. Also, e-learning can be more effective than printed learning materials for reducing stigma and disability from mental illness. Training trainers in MHFA is also an effective way to increase the use, dissemination, and application of information as well as improve mental health literacy (Jorm, et al., 2010).

MHFA has five steps. The first step is to assess the risk of suicide or harm to an individual. The second step is to listen nonjudgmentally to the individual seeking support. The third step is to provide reassurance and information to the distressed person or group. The fourth step is to provide encouragement to the distressed person/group and to obtain appropriate professional assistance. The fifth step is to encourage self-help strategies for the distressed individual/group (Kitchener & Jorm, 2006). Research has demonstrated that through MHFA training, a whole community can provide aid through formal mental health services with early identification and intervention of mental illness (Kitchener & Jorm, 2008).

Solution-Focused Therapy

An effective form of mental health treatment is solution-focused therapy. This can be applied through psychoeducation, mental health first aid, and training efforts to support large-scale interventions. Solution-focused therapy focuses on the strengths individuals already possess and the belief that people already have the resources they need to solve their own problems. A growing body of evidence for this therapy approach exists, and many applications can be potentially incorporated into mental health literacy literature and mental health first aid interventions (Corcoran & Pillai, 2009). Solution-focused brief therapy (SFBT) is a future-focused, goal-oriented brief therapy. SFBT is developed from practical observations. It is an approach that focuses on identifying what is working in relationships and situations and building on that. An important distinction of SFBT is its focus and language on solutions, not on problems (De Shazer et al., 2021).

The language of problems is different from the language and perspective of solutions. Some central components of SFBT are that (1) if something works, do more of it, (2) if something is not broken, don't change it, (3) if it's not working, do something different, (4) small steps can result in big changes, (5) solutions are not necessarily directed related to the problem, (6) look for exceptions in the problem, no problems happen all the time, and (7) the future is not known; it is created and flexible. Solution-focused therapy is a highly successful, popular, and extensively used therapy. It is grounded in pragmatism, resiliency, and a client's own history of solutions and exceptions to problems. SFBT works to build on an individual's strengths and resiliencies, helps them identify these aspects, and increases those behaviors. This approach is positively future-focused and can be applied in a mental health first aid and psychoeducational format (De Shazer et al., 2021).

Cognitive Behavior Therapy

Another important approach for mental health treatment in the future is cognitive behavioral therapy (CBT). This is a well-known, evidence-based approach that is widely used with psychoeducation and traditional therapy. CBT has been found to positively impact substance use disorders, schizophrenia, psychosis, depression, mood disorder, anxiety disorder, bipolar disorder, eating disorder, insomnia, personality disorder, anger, criminal behavior, stress, chronic pain and fatigue, distress related to medical conditions, and more. CBT is a very strong evidence-based approach. It is used worldwide and supported by many government-sponsored mental health initiatives like in the United Kingdom (Hofmann et al., 2012).

CBT has been integrated into even more effective, evidence-based approaches with the growth of mindfulness-based treatments and acceptance and commitment therapy (ACT). Mindfulness-based treatments focus on a present-moment, nonjudgmental approach. Dialectical behavior therapy (DBT) is an evidence-based intervention and a derivative of CBT that combines structured mindfulness-based techniques with acceptance and change as a central component for emotional regulation. DBT emphasizes acceptance, emotional distress tolerance, and insight into cognitions, emotions, and behaviors (Hofmann et al., 2010).

A way to increasingly implement these approaches is via e-mental health. E-mental health refers to mental health services and information delivered or enhanced through the Internet and related technology. Mobile health apps offering e-mental health are effective for mental health interventions alongside CBT. E-mental health is an effective way to provide support for individuals with mental illness and limited resources (Denecke et al., 2022).

Rational Emotive Behavior Therapy

Rational emotive behavior therapy (REBT) is an effective approach that focuses on irrational and rational beliefs. It helps individuals to change irrational beliefs to rational beliefs to better cope with reality and difficult circumstances. ACT, CBT, and REBT are all evidence-based approaches with greater application worldwide through psychoeducation, group therapy, government-supported interventions, and clinical therapeutic practice (DiGiuseppe & David, 2015). REBT is psychoeducational because it believes that individuals can be taught skills to identify, challenge, and replace dysfunctional beliefs on their own. It provides an opportunity for larger, global mental health workers because of the psychoeducational emphasis on resiliency and flexibility (Jordana et al., 2020).

Group Support and Group Therapy

Another important component of future happiness and well-being treatment is group therapy, group support, and group psychoeducation, both online and in person. This provides a format to deliver information, impact larger numbers of people, and help an individual facilitator serve a greater number of clients. This platform can be effective in helping individuals learn from other group members, learn skills to function effectively and manage negative emotions (Berg et al., 2017). Group counseling can also be used preventatively to teach self-help mechanisms such as REBT, mindfulness, self-compassion, and other teachable tools. Preventive group psychoeducational therapy can be a useful approach to help individuals and also potentially bypass concerns regarding mental health literacy and stigma (Berg et al., 2017).

Yoga

Yoga is an increasingly important complementary and alternative medical treatment for mental health disorders. Complementary and alternative medicine can be effective in providing mental health support in areas of mental health stigma, mental health illiteracy, and resource-poor regions, where paying for mental health services is not viable. Yoga is considered a type of complementary and alternative medical treatment and has been used for thousands of years for good physical and mental health. Yoga can be applied for prevention, health promotion, and also for support mental health disorders (Gangadhar & Varambally, 2011).

Family Therapy

Family therapy looks at relational difficulties among family members and also systems. This approach can be helpful and impact mental health literacy and stigma. Family therapy and systems therapy is a growing approach that goes beyond traditional individual therapeutic practices. It can be worthwhile to consider future applications of this modality in other cultures and how it can be used in a larger way (Carr, 2012).

Latin America and E-Health

Internet-based interventions for the prevention and management of mental illness are rapidly growing in Latin America (Jiménez-Molina et al., 2019). Studies conducted on telehealth treatment in Brazil, Mexico, Colombia, and Chile for depression achieved similar positive outcomes in symptom reduction as traditional face-to-face in-person treatment. Internet-based self-help programs are initially useful, but adherence and completion rates tend to be low (Jiménez-Molina et al., 2019). Telehealth therapy and psychiatry interventions may be an effective way to increase outpatient mental health treatment and reduce depression in a low-cost, easy-to-implement manner. Psychoeducational programs conducted in Brazil and Peru using mobile phones found increases in daily life activities, motivation, education on self-care, and reduction in depression symptoms as a result of mobile phone programs. Smartphones may be a positive and effective alternative for accessing teletherapy support (Jiménez-Molina et al., 2019). Internet and digital technologies improve access to and create greater flexibility for mental health treatment (Jiménez-Molina et al., 2019). Tele-mental health is a way to reach people who would otherwise not access mental healthcare due to physical limitations or stigma. Providers based remotely outside communities through telehealth can provide a sense of safety to be open and seek treatment (Phillip, 2017). Tele-mental health is a potential major solution for treatment and can be accessed by much larger numbers of people in Latin America, thereby addressing a significant public health concern (Phillip, 2017).

Prevention

Another component of mental healthcare is not only early treatment and interventions but also prevention. By preventing the main risk factors that lead to mental illness, we can reduce the overall burden on society and the need to significantly expand treatment. The individual attributes that put one at risk for mental illness include low self-esteem, emotional immaturity, trouble with communication, medical illness, and substance abuse. Social circumstances that put one at risk for mental illness include loneliness, bereavement, neglect, family conflict, exposure to violence/abuse, low income and poverty, difficulties or failure at school, and work stress or unemployment. Environmental factors that significantly impact mental health include poor access to basic services, injustice and discrimination, and exposure to war or disaster. Any or all combinations of these can lead to the development of mental illness in an individual (Helliwell & Wang, 2013; Helliwell et al., 2013; Layard et al., 2013).

Early intervention programs and mental health initiatives serve as protective or preventive factors in developing mental illness. Interventions that are implemented in home, work, community, and school-based environments are effective for addressing needs. The stigma and misunderstanding about mental health may preclude individuals from accessing or trying to access mental health services. Psychosocial support through education and public health measures may be effective for addressing variables that put an individual at risk of mental illness and also for learning how to manage early symptoms (Helliwell & Wang, 2013; Helliwell et al., 2013; Layard et al., 2013).

CONCLUSION

This chapter discusses multiple components of the future of mental health and wellness globally. Concerns such as mental health stigma, mental health literacy, and mental health first aid are examined. Effective approaches for the future of mental health treatment are explored such as solution-focused therapy, rational emotive behavior therapy, group therapy, cognitive behavior therapy, family therapy, and complementary approaches such as yoga. The relevancy of e-health, psychoeducation, and public health campaigns is also explored.

LIST OF KEY TAKEAWAYS

- Mental health concerns are rising in importance worldwide.
- The future of mental health necessitates large-scale, low-cost interventions that can bypass mental health illiteracy, accessibility, cost, and stigma concerns.
- E-health and mobile devices provide an important mechanism to address current and future mental health needs.
- There is a major need to implement large-scale, effective, low-cost interventions for the future of mental health.

REVIEW QUESTIONS

- What are the general global trends for mental health in the future?
- What surprised you about this chapter?
- If you could create an intervention to support future mental health needs, what would you create?
- What are some potential positive approaches for the future with mental health?

REFERENCES

Berg, R. C., Landreth, G. L., & Fall, K. A. (2017). *Group counseling: Concepts and procedures.* Routledge.

Bharadwaj, P., Pai, M. M., & Suziedelyte, A. (2017). Mental health stigma. *Economics Letters, 159,* 5760. https://doi.org/10.1016/j.econlet.2017.06.028

Carr, A. (2012). *Family therapy: Concepts, process and practice.* John Wiley & Sons.

Corcoran, J., & Pillai, V. (2009). A review of the research on solution-focused therapy. *British Journal of Social Work, 39*(2), 234–242. https://doi.org/10.1093/bjsw/bcm098

Denecke, K., Schmid, N., & Nüssli, S. (2022). Implementation of cognitive behavioral therapy in e–mental health apps: Literature review. *Journal of Medical Internet Research, 24*(3), e27791. https://doi.org/10.2196/27791

De Shazer, S., Dolan, Y., Korman, H., Trepper, T., McCollum, E., & Berg, I. K. (2021). *More than miracles: The state of the art of solution-focused brief therapy.* Routledge.

DiGiuseppe, R., & David, O. A. (2015). Rational emotive behavior therapy. In H. T. Prout & A. L. Fedewa (Eds.), *Counseling and psychotherapy with children and adolescents: Theory and practice for school and clinical settings* (pp. 155–215). John Wiley & Sons Inc.

Ganasen, K. A., Parker, S., Hugo, C. J., Stein, D. J., Emsley, R. A., & Seedat, S. (2008). Mental health literacy: Focus on developing countries. *African Journal of Psychiatry, 11*(1), 23–28. https://doi.org/10.4314/ajpsy.v11i1.30251

Gangadhar, B. N., & Varambally, S. (2011). Yoga as therapy in psychiatric disorders: Past, present, and future. *Biofeedback, 39*(2), 60–63. https://doi.org/10.5298/1081-5937-39.2.03

Helliwell, J. F., Layard, R., & Sachs, J. (Eds.) (2013). *World happiness report 2013.* Sustainable Development Solutions Network. *https://worldhappiness.report/ed/2013/*

Helliwell, J. F., Layard, R., & Sachs, J. (Eds.) (2015). *World happiness report 2015.* Sustainable Development Solutions Network. https://worldhappiness.report/ed/2015/

Helliwell, J. F., & Wang, S. (2013). World happiness: Trends, explanations and distribution. In J. Helliwell, R. Layard, & J. Sachs (Eds.), *World happiness report 2013. Sustainable Development Solutions Network. https://worldhappiness.report/ed/2013/*

Hofmann, S. G., Asnaani, A., Vonk, I. J., Sawyer, A. T., & Fang, A. (2012). The efficacy of cognitive behavioral therapy: A review of meta-analyses. *Cognitive Therapy and Research, 36,* 427–440. https://doi.org/10.1007/s10608-012-9476-1

Hofmann, S. G., Sawyer, A. T., & Fang, A. (2010). The empirical status of the "new wave" of cognitive behavioral therapy. *Psychiatric Clinics, 33*(3), 701–710. https://doi.org/10.1016/j.psc.2010.04.006

Jiménez-Molina, Á., Franco, P., Martínez, V., Martínez, P., Rojas, G., & Araya, R. (2019). Internet-based interventions for the prevention and treatment of mental disorders in Latin America: A scoping review. *Frontiers in Psychiatry, 10*(664). https://doi.org/10.3389/fpsyt.2019.00664

Jordana, A., Turner, M. J., Ramis, Y., & Torregrossa, M. (2020). A systematic mapping review on the use of rational emotive behavior therapy (REBT) with athletes. *International Review of Sport and Exercise Psychology,* 1–26. https://doi.org/10.1080/1750984X.2020.1836673

Jorm, A. F., Kitchener, B. A., Fischer, J. A., & Cvetkovski, S. (2010). Mental health first aid training by e-learning: A randomized controlled trial. *Australian & New Zealand Journal of Psychiatry, 44*(12), 1072–1081. https://doi.org/10.3109/00048674.2010.516426

Kelly, C. M., Jorm, A. F., & Wright, A. (2007). Improving mental health literacy as a strategy to facilitate early intervention for mental disorders. *Medical Journal of Australia, 187*(S7), S26–S30. https://doi.org/10.5694/j.1326-5377.2007.tb01332.x

Kitchener, B. A., & Jorm, A. F. (2006). Mental health first aid training: Review of evaluation studies. *Australian & New Zealand Journal of Psychiatry, 40*(1), 68. https://doi.org/10.1080/j.1440-1614.2006.01735.x

Kitchener, B. A., & Jorm, A. F. (2008). Mental health first aid: An international programme for early intervention. *Early Intervention in Psychiatry, 2*(1), 55–61. https://doi.org/10.1111/j.1751-7893.2007.00056.x

Layard, R., Chisholm, D., Patel, V., & Saxena, S. (2013). Mental illness and unhappiness. (Discussion Paper No. 1239) Center for Economic Performance, London School of Economics and Political Science. https://cep.lse.ac.uk/pubs/download/dp1239.pdf

Layard, R., & Hagell, A. (2015). Healthy young minds: Transforming the mental health of children. In J. F. Helliwell, R. Layard, & J. Sachs (Eds.), *World happiness report (pp.* 106–131). Sustainable Development Solutions Network. https://worldhappiness. report/ed/2015/

Phillip, T. M. (2017). Telemental health in Latin America and the Caribbean. In H. Jefee-Bahloul, A. Barkil-Oteo, & E. G. Augusterfer (Eds.), *Telemental health in resource-limited global settings (pp.* 181–192). *Oxford University Press.*

Sickel, A. E., Seacat, J. D., & Nabors, N. A. (2014). Mental health stigma update: A review of consequences. *Advances in Mental Health, 12(*3), 202–215. https://doi.org/10.1080/18374905.2014.11081898

www.ingramcontent.com/pod-product-compliance
Lightning Source LLC
Chambersburg PA
CBHW042339030426
42335CB00030B/3400

9781964097565